Strategies for National Quality and Payment Policy

Guest Editors

NANCY GIRARD, PhD, RN, FAAN
MICKEY PARSONS, PhD, RN, FAAN

PERIOPERATIVE NURSING CLINICS

www.periopnursing.theclinics.com

September 2012 • Volume 7 • Number 3

SAUNDERS an imprint of ELSEVIER, Inc.

W.B. SAUNDERS COMPANY

A Division of Elsevier Inc.

1600 John F. Kennedy Boulevard • Suite 1800 • Philadelphia, Pennsylvania 19103-2899

http://www.periopnursing.theclinics.com

PERIOPERATIVE NURSING CLINICS Volume 7, Number 3
September 2012 ISSN 1556-7931, ISBN-13: 978-1-4557-4909-6

Editor: Katie Hartner
Developmental Editor: Donald Mumford

Perioperative Nursing Clinics (ISSN 1556-7931) is published quarterly by Elsevier, 360 Park Avenue South, New York, NY 10010. Months of issue are March, June, September and December. Business and Editorial Offices: 1600 John F. Kennedy Blvd., Suite 1800, Philadelphia, PA 19103-2899. Customer Service Office: 11830 Westline Industrial Drive, St. Louis, MO 63146. Periodicals postage paid at New York, NY and at additional mailing offices. Subscription prices are $132.00 per year (domestic individuals), $224.00 per year (domestic institutions), $65.00.00 per year (domestic students/ residents), $171.00 per year (international individuals), $257.00 per year (international institutions), and $69.00 per year (International students/residents). Foreign air speed delivery is included in all *Clinics* subscription prices. All prices are subject to change without notice. **POSTMASTER:** Send change of address to *Perioperative Nursing Clinics,* Customer Service (orders, claims, online, change of address): Elsevier Periodicals Customer Service, 11830 Westline Industrial Drive, St. Louis, MO 63146. Tel: 1-800-654-2452 (U.S. and Canada). Fax: 314-523-5170. E-mail: journalscustomerservice-usa@elsevier.com (for print support); journalsonlinesupport-usa@elsevier.com (for online support).

Reprints. For copies of 100 or more, of articles in this publication, please contact the Commercial Rights Department, Elsevier Inc., 360 Park Avenue South, New York, NY 10010-1710; Phone: (+1) 212-633-3813; Fax: (+1) 212-462-1935; E-mail: reprints@elsevier.com.

Printed and bound by CPI Group (UK) Ltd, Croydon, CR0 4YY

Transferred to Digital Print 2012

Contributors

CONSULTING EDITOR

NANCY GIRARD, PhD, RN, FAAN
Nurse Collaborations, Boerne, Texas; Clinical Associate Professor, Acute Nursing Care Department, University of Texas Health Science Center, San Antonio, Texas

GUEST EDITORS

NANCY GIRARD, PhD, RN, FAAN
Nurse Collaborations, Boerne, Texas; Clinical Associate Professor, Acute Nursing Care Department, University of Texas Health Science Center, San Antonio, Texas

MICKEY PARSONS, PhD, MHA, RN, FAAN
Howard & Betty Halff Professor for Excellence in Patient Care, UT Health Science Center, San Antonio School of Nursing, San Antonio, Texas

AUTHORS

GRETCHEL AJON-GEALOGO, MSN, RN-BC, CMSRN
Doctoral Student, School of Nursing, University of Texas Health Science Center at San Antonio, San Antonio, Texas

ANDREA E. BERNDT, PhD
School of Nursing, University of Texas Health Science Center at San Antonio

DEBORAH CARVER, MSN, RN
University of Texas Health Science Center, San Antonio, Austin, Texas

PATRICIA A. CORNETT, EdD, MS, RN
CEO, Solúcion Associates, LCC, Canyon Lake, Texas; Adjunct Associate Professor, Graduate Administration Program, School of Nursing, University of Texas Health Science Center at San Antonio, San Antonio, Texas

CLARICE GOLIGHTLY-JENKINS, PhD, MSN, RN, CNS
Methodist Healthcare System, San Antonio, Texas

JACQUELINE M. GORDON, MSN, RN, CCNS, CCRN
Clinical Nurse Specialist, Heart and Vascular Institute, Penn State Hershey Medical Center, Hershey, Pennsylvania

CHERYL A. LEHMAN, PhD, RN, CNS-BC, RN-BC, CRRN
Clinical Associate Professor, Department of Health Restoration and Care Systems Management, School of Nursing, University of Texas Health Science Center at San Antonio, San Antonio, Texas

MAJ JENNIFER D. LORILLA, MSN, RN, United States Army Nurse Corps
Clinical Nurse Specialist, Department of Medicine, Tripler Army Medical Center, Hawaii

MICKEY PARSONS, PhD, MHA, RN, FAAN
Howard & Betty Halff Professor for Excellence in Patient Care School of Nursing,
University of Texas Health Science Center at San Antonio, San Antonio, Texas

CYNTHIA VORPAHL PURCELL, MSN, RN
Clinical Assistant Professor, Department of Health Restoration and Care Systems
Management, School of Nursing, University of Texas Health Science Center at
San Antonio, San Antonio, Texas; DNP program, University of Alabama,
Birmingham, Alabama

CATHERINE ROBICHAUX, PhD, RN, CCRN, CNS
Faculty Associate, Department of Health Restoration and Systems Care Management,
University of Texas Health Science Center, San Antonio, Texas

JEANIE SAUERLAND, BS, BSN, RN
Nurse Educator, PACU, OPS, UPOMC, Chair, Nursing Ethics Committee, University
Health System, San Antonio, Texas

Contents

In fiscal year 2013, value-based purchasing will be implemented. A portion of Medicare payments for hospital stays will be determined by performance and comparison with other facilities. Reimbursement will be at risk as the threshold is adjusted upward. Providers must strive to improve patient satisfaction and quality measures to remain competitive, ensure eligibility for pay incentives, and maintain (if applicable) Magnet status. This article describes a relationship-based care model for addressing patient satisfaction. In these difficult financial times, the implementation strategies for a practice model must have a minimal impact financially. This approach facilitates change within teams and cultures.

Individuals in middle management positions in the twenty-first century can optimize their clinical care system through use of a leader practice framework that integrates a focus on people with an evidence-based approach to empower and energize those at the frontline of health care who deliver the care and services to patients. The interplay of the 5 functions in the Positional Leadership Framework provides a unifying road map for optimizing microsystems.

This article describes the development, implementation, and preliminary evaluation of the Interprofessional Study Group for Quality Improvement (ISG) at a multihospital metropolitan tertiary health system. Participants read chapters and facilitated weekly discussions using a text in the Dartmouth Quality Improvement Curriculum, interviewed patients about their hospital experiences, identified care gaps from interview data, and presented a pilot plan for a quality improvement initiative. Although few differences were noted between pre and post responses, participants' comments about shared learning with a common language, and learning from patient interviews suggest the approach facilitated interest, enthusiasm, and intent to collaborate in future initiatives.

Frontline nurses need to understand how they impact national patient care quality measures and benchmarks. For perioperative nurses, the Surgical

Care Improvement Project (SCIP) process measures in the Joint Commission's Core Measures Data Set dictate current evidence-based standards of care. This article (1) provides the rationale for using primers and dashboards as tools for disseminating and incorporating SCIP into frontline perioperative nursing practice, (2) introduces Knowles' and Vygotsky's learning theories to provide complementary perspectives on the nature of adult learning, and (3) outlines teaching strategies and exemplars that may be used to evaluate learner progress.

This article proposes that ethics is the framework that supports quality and that nurses are central in this interdependence. A brief history of the nursing profession's concern with quality and ethics is presented. A discussion of ethical principles, virtue ethics, and the ethics of care is provided. Implications of the principles and virtue/care approaches for practice and leadership and their impact on quality care are suggested. An example of ongoing collaboration between staff nurses and leadership to improve quality care through development of a nursing ethics council and unit-based ethics steward program is presented.

The Clinical Nurse Specialist (CNS) has often struggled with attaining recognition, reimbursement, and regard as an Advanced Practice Registered Nurse (APRN). Some markets limit the CNS to a single role (typically, the nurse educator), whereas others use the CNS to their fullest potential as clinical expert, involving their CNS employees in quality monitoring and improvement, implementation of evidence-based practices in the workplace, and as expert clinical practitioners in varied settings including primary, secondary, and tertiary care. This article explores the future of the CNS in health care in the United States.

The Texas Public Policy Foundation is a nonprofit, nonpartisan research organization providing credible and valuable information that nurses can use in their pursuits to influence health care policy. The information is rich and is produced in such a way that the general public can understand the issues as well as the impact of pending and future legislation. The Foundation's publications are excellent resources for nurses practicing in Texas and around the nation. As the Director of the Center for Health Care Policy at the Foundation, Arlene Wohlgemuth is an accessible and approachable resource and friend to nurses.

PERIOPERATIVE NURSING CLINICS

**Perioperative Nursing Clinics will cease publication
with the December 2012 issue**

NOW AVAILABLE FOR YOUR iPhone and iPad

Preface

Changing Policy and Nursing Strategies

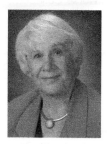 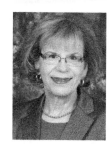

Nancy Girard, PhD, RN, FAAN   Mickey Parsons, PhD, RN, FAAN
Guest Editors

Do all nurses need to understand policy and its impact on patient care and the profession? Yes, indeed! A fundamental understanding of policy is essential for both understanding current trends in health care and for deriving an effective approach to government, provider, and educational organizations. At both federal and state levels, policy drives legislation. Legislation determines programs and impacts associated funding for specific patient care activities. It also affects educational and research activities that can expand the nursing profession to meet society's needs better. Thus, the purpose of this issue is to provide the reader with a broad perspective of the numerous policy issues with which we are confronted in today's health care workplace, and to provide selected strategies that will assist nurses in working with legislators in forming policies that will impact health care for all patients.

Within this issue, Cornett presents the reader with a comprehensive professional practice framework for the successful delivery of nursing care in the new era of transparency and nursing's responsibility for outcomes in the processes of care. Carver and Parsons summarize value-based purchasing and offer a strategy to improve the patient's experience. Gealogo presents a primer to teach nurses how to utilize dashboards that will allow them to understand outcome indicators better for designing practice improvement initiatives.

The implications for practice and education, incorporating the public mandate for quality care, are further explicated by Kendall-Gallagher. Robichaux and colleagues discuss the implications of ethics and practice. An innovative pilot study to educate the leaders for quality and nursing staff development, along with additional key members of the interprofessional team, is also reported for one organization's strategy to fulfill its obligation to society to provide quality care and outcomes. Last, Gordon and her coauthors present the educational and policy question of the role of the Clinical

Perioperative Nursing Clinics 7 (2012) ix–x
http://dx.doi.org/10.1016/j.cpen.2012.06.008   **periopnursing.theclinics.com**

Nurse Specialist, and Purcell summarizes an interview of a prominent leader in a health policy foundation.

We thank all the wonderful contributors to this issue and hope you, the reader, find this issue informative and useful.

Nancy Girard, PhD, RN, FAAN
Nurse Collaborations
Boerne, TX

Mickey Parsons, PhD, RN, FAAN
The University of Texas Health
Science Center at San Antonio
School of Nursing
San Antonio, TX, USA

E-mail addresses:
ngirard2@satx.rr.com (N. Girard)
parsonsm@uthscsa.edu (M. Parsons)

Value-Based Purchasing and Practice Strategies

Deborah Carver, MSN, RN*, Mickey Parsons, PhD, MHA, RN, FAAN

KEYWORDS

- Hospital value-based purchasing • HCAHPS • Practice strategies
- Relationship-Based Care

KEY POINTS

- It is vital that patient satisfaction remains a focus for every hospital. As all hospitals work to improve patient satisfaction scores, the fiftieth percentile is sure to increase.
- The culture change resulting from the implementation of professional practice model strengthens the team and the care provided.
- The suggested grassroots approach facilitates change from within the individual units and provides a way forward to achieve lasting culture change.

INTRODUCTION

The ever-rising health care costs in the United States are driving significant changes in policy and practice. One of those primary changes was the Affordable Care Act of 2010. This act established the Hospital Value-Based Purchasing (VBP) program under the Medicare Inpatient Prospective Payment System designed to promote higher quality patient care in hospitals. The program does not include inpatient stays at rehabilitation, psychiatric, long-term care, children's, or cancer hospitals.[1] Starting in fiscal year 2013, a portion of Medicare payments for inpatient stays will be determined by performance scores of several quality measures. The quality measures are broken out into 12 clinical process measures (70% of the total score) and 8 patient experience measures evaluated by the Hospital Consumer Assessment of Healthcare Providers and Systems (HCAHPS) survey (30% of the total score).[1] The clinical process measures can be seen in **Box 1** along with a deeper explanation of HCAHPS scores. In fiscal year 2014, CMS will add mortality outcome measures for myocardial infarction, heart failure, and pneumonia.[1]

Specifically, hospitals will experience a 1% reduction in Medicare reimbursement in fiscal year 2013. The dollars the government holds back will go into a fund from which hospitals will be paid a dollar amount based on how their final score compares to other

UT Health Science Center, San Antonio School of Nursing, 7703 Floyd Curl Drive, San Antonio, TX 78229-3900, USA
* Corresponding author.
E-mail address: carverd@livemail.uthscsa.edu

Perioperative Nursing Clinics 7 (2012) 297–303
http://dx.doi.org/10.1016/j.cpen.2012.06.005
1556-7931/12/$ – see front matter © 2012 Elsevier Inc. All rights reserved.

Box 1
Clinical process of care measures table

Acute myocardial infarction

Fibrinolytic therapy received within 30 minutes of hospital arrival

Primary percutaneous coronary intervention received within 90 minutes of hospital arrival

Heart failure

Discharge instructions

Pneumonia

Blood cultures performed in the emergency department before initial antibiotic received in hospital

Initial antibiotic selection for community-acquired pneumonia in immunocompetent patient

Healthcare-associated infections

Prophylactic antibiotic received within 1 hour before surgical incision

Prophylactic antibiotic selection for surgical patients

Prophylactic antibiotics discontinued within 24 hours after surgery end time

Cardiac surgery patients with controlled 6:00 AM postoperative serum glucose

surgeries

Surgery patients on a beta blocker before arrival who received a beta blocker during the perioperative period

Surgery patients with recommended venous thromboembolism prophylaxis ordered

Surgery patients who received appropriate venous thromboembolism prophylaxis within 24 hours before surgery to 24 hours after surgery

From Department of Health and Human Services. Medicare Program. Hospital Inpatient Value-Based Purchasing Program. 2011. Available at: http://www.gpo.gov/fdsys/pkg/FR-2011-05-06/pdf/2011-10568.pdf.

hospitals participating in the program. Those hospitals that achieve the highest score will receive the largest incentive payment and those at the lower end of the spectrum will lose reimbursement. Furthermore, to increasingly fund the VBP dollar pool for incentive payments, Medicare cuts will increase each year by 0.25% until 2017.[1] Given the dramatic landscape change and the associated public demand for quality care, this article focuses on strategies to improve the patient experience.

STRATEGY: HOW TO IMPROVE HCAHPS SCORES

There is much debate about how to improve and maintain HCAHPS scores. Some clinicians may argue that a health care organization should focus on all components of HCAHPS questions because 20 of the 100 eligible points for the patient experience in VBP is derived from a consistency calculation that rewards hospitals that achieve at least the median score in each area.[2] However, resourcing a broad-based strategy plan may be prohibitive in today's economic environment and, therefore, unrealistic. Professional Research Consultants (PRC), a company that performs patient-experience telephone surveys, suggests focusing on the areas that require the smallest increase to achieve additional points.[3] However, the area of focus may be different for each clinical area and vary month to month. Success will depend on the strength of the frontline leader. It is suggested that an overarching targeted focus guide clinicians' to improve HCAHPS scores. In this article, the focus is improving caregiver communication and teamwork.

THE RELATIONSHIP-BASED CARE MODEL

What methodology might a health care organization select to focus on caregiver communication and teamwork? A professional practice model, such as Relationship-Based Care (RBC), is suggested because of its strong emphasis on communication, which guides the creation of satisfying relationships at multiple levels. A professional-practice model is defined by Hoffart and Woods[4] as "system (structure, process, and values) that supports registered nurse control over the delivery of nursing care and the environment in which care is delivered." The RBC practice model is formed by the concept of caring and focuses on three relationships: between caregiver and patient and family, between team members, and with self.[5] "Studies demonstrate a positive impact from the implementation of models of caring with regard to the work environment of nursing, retention, nurse and patient satisfaction, and patient outcomes."[6] Additionally, for a hospital on the journey for recognition as a Magnet hospital or redesignation, a practice model is a requirement because it is the foundation for best practice in nursing care. The RBC practice model centers on the patient and family in all aspects of care delivery and the positive impact has been demonstrated in numerous organizations. For example, Michigan Mercy Hospital reported a 5% increase in the overall rating of care[7] and St. Mary's Medical Center, a large nonprofit hospital in Evansville, Indiana, demonstrated an increase from a low of 8.5 for patient satisfaction before implementation to 9.02 after implementation of RBC on a 10-point scale.[6]

To further describe the RBC model, the theoretical underpinnings from caring theory are depicted. Watson's Theory of Human Caring, Swanson's Theory of Caring, and Dingman's Caring Model all form the RBC framework.[5] At their core, all the theories value the nurse-to-patient relationship. In Watson's theory, "caring-healing modalities and nursing arts are reintegrated as essentials to ensure attention to quality of life, inner healing experiences, subjective meaning, and caring practices, which affect both patient outcomes and system success. It is this human-to-human caring that is central to the professional nurse's practice and responsibility."[8] According to Swanson, the five processes of caring are knowing, being with, doing for, enabling, and maintaining belief.[9] The nurse's "... work integrates caring and healing consciousness with nurse behaviors and speaks directly to the elements of RBC."[10] Dingman's contribution is a model to apply the theories. In an evaluation of the implementation of the five specific caring behaviors, a positive impact on patient satisfaction of a 9% percent improvement in overall satisfaction was found.[5]

STRATEGY SPECIFICS

Implementing RBC is a valuable method to address the challenges in VBP and creating a culture of caring in an organization. Successful implementation could protect generic reimbursement rates and position the facility to receive incentive monies as competition increases and funding decreases overall. Using the expertise of consultants to guide and educate the staff could be the easiest approach for introducing RBC into a facility. However, this can be very costly. Senior executives must weigh the costs versus benefits and may find that in these tight economic times funding this new initiative could prove to be difficult. Many facilities are experiencing a shift in payer mix, with a decline in the private insurer and an increase in Medicaid and

Medicare patients. There are also competing priorities for funding, whether it is for developing a new service line, ensuring regulatory compliance, or improvements in training and retention. Thus, an executive and middle management team that values developing a culture of caring relationships as the overarching strategy must create a proposal targeted to attaining maximum direct care impact and HCAHPS scores for a minimum expenditure.

KOTTER'S EIGHT-STEP CHANGE MODEL GUIDES IMPLEMENTATION

The following is an example of a grassroots approach that could be adopted for any clinical area based on their patient population and services. In hospitals already engaged in shared governance, a bottom up approach to implementing RBC can provide a low-cost avenue for a new initiative. Through shared governance, the concept of RBC may be introduced to the staff at multiple levels. A management and staff RBC steering committee provides structure and support for the unit councils and, through staff facilitation at unit councils, the caregivers identify specific changes in provider-to-provider communication and team work.

A structured, yet facilitated, approach is needed for organizational success. Given that there are many models for change, using a well studied model in the business world, such as Kotter's eight-step change model, facilitates the culture-change process essential to effective implementation of RBC.[11] The model is straightforward and provides an easy-to-follow framework in which success is measured by the engagement and buy-in of the employees. Using Kotter's change model, implementation steps for RBC are as follows[12]:

- Step 1: Establishing a sense of urgency
  - Identify a project leader. Strong leadership is necessary to champion this transformation. To provide the project leader with a foundation for RBC, a useful first step includes reading and becoming informed about RBC and caring theories. There are multiple books on the RBC and consulting companies that provide in depth training and consultation services.
  - Further develop facility steering committee and unit council leader's and educators' knowledge of HCAHPS (linking HCAHPS to quality and safety), VBP, and RBC.
    - Project leader develops and provides a presentation that relates core measures, HCAHPS, and VBP to the facility's nursing leadership team.
- Step 2: Creating the guiding coalition
  - Establish a learning community, such as an "RBC Book Club," with unit leaders and educators.
  - From the learning community, RBC Book Club group creates a steering committee to oversee the transformation, if it was not formerly established.
- Step 3: Developing a change vision
  - The Book Club members develop a specific change vision for RBC to affect the facility culture for caring relationships. Specific caring behaviors in practice are identified and strategies developed to achieve them. Dingman's Caring Model and specific behaviors contribute to the examples of the vision, which are:
    - "Introduce yourself to the patient and explain your role in their care that day
    - Call the patient by his or her preferred name
    - Sit at the patient's bedside for at least 5 minutes per shift to plan and review the patient's care
    - Use a handshake, or touch on the arm
    - Use the mission, vision, and value statements in planning your care."[13]

- Begin work to integrate RBC into the hospital and unit goals.
- Work with the human resources leaders to review job descriptions and evaluation process to ensure that relationship based care is integrated.
- Incorporate RBC into new-hire patient-loyalty training.
- Leaders and educators further design frontline training and "toolboxes" to support unit councils.

- Step 4: Communicating the vision for buy-in
  - Expand the RBC Book Clubs to all units and invite key interprofessional (ancillary, support staff) to participate at the microsystem level.
  - Expand educational tools to include online education with voiceover to introduce Relationship-Based Care and the Caring Model to all frontline staff to further establish a sense of urgency and communicate the vision.
  - Place articles about RBC in the hospital newsletters.
  - Provide articles for unit-level newsletters.
  - Use the marketing department to help create promotional materials.

- Step 5: Empowering broad-based action
  - Charge and empower unit-based councils to lead the change and insure that one of the registered nurse champions is the unit-based council chair.
  - The overall project leader, now identified as the project coordinator, meets with the unit-level managers and educator to assess their level of engagement and support the reduction of barriers and amplification of facilitators.
  - Encourage council leads, educators, and leadership to participate in additional staff development as it is offered through the hospital's organizational development department.
    - Hold a change-management class.
    - Hold a class on how to run effective meetings.
  - Provide an initial 4-hour unit retreat through an expanded unit-level council meeting time. Review lessons learned to-date, determine any additional information that may be needed for the team, and develop a unit-specific vision and practice specifics in each clinical area. The project coordinator shares tools and suggestions, helps identify system issues that may undermine the vision, and takes any barriers to change back to the leadership for discussion.
    - Use IDEA model (Investigate, Design, Execute, Adjust).
    - Monitor results.

- Step 6: Generating short-term wins
  - Unit-level councils continue over the next several months with a focus on RBC to create improvements.
    - Facility leader and steering committee supports units in the revision of their unit scope of service to include RBC.
    - Identify an initial teamwork development strategy through developing a Commitment to Coworkers document.
    - Set goals for individual HCAHPS scores.
    - Facility leader and steering committee monitors progress and creates rewards and recognition for improvements.

- Step 7: Never letting up
  - Unit managers continue to support the focus by hiring only potential staff who support the vision and caring practices, and promote and support unit leaders, both formally and informally, to drive progress.
  - Unit managers demonstrate the organization's priority for RBC through intentional unit rounds and observation. This sends a clear message of expected staff behaviors. It also provides the manager an opportunity to give both

positive and constructive feedback in real time that contributes to accountability and staff problem solving.
- Institute daily stand-up huddles.
- Unit-level council incorporates PRC data review into monthly meetings and posts for all staff.
- Senior leadership support the steering committee, unit councils, and focus follow-up on areas with highest percent of discharges related to HCAHPS.
- Step 8: Incorporating changes into the culture
  - Hold follow-up discussions in unit meetings to demonstrate that new behaviors are affecting results.
  - Continue to offer leadership development opportunities.

With a thoughtful structured approach and using a grassroots shared governance process, Kotter's Eight-Step Change model provides a useful guide for transformation of a facility's culture for caring relationships, and improving communication and teamwork. The intent of this approach is to imbed caring behaviors into the work of all staff to ultimately improve HCAHPS results. It does demand a hard-working, creative, and dedicated leader and team. However, engaging the staff early in the process and using their skills and talents will lead to lasting change.

SUMMARY

It is vital that patient satisfaction remains a focus for every hospital. As all hospitals work to improve patient satisfaction scores, the fiftieth percentile is sure to increase. Magnet hospitals must stay above the fiftieth percentile to maintain the Magnet status and the loss of Magnet designation would have a profound negative impact on an organization. In addition, a lack of focus on HCAHPS results can culminate in a loss of funds from Medicare based on VBP. More importantly, the improvement efforts required of VBP are not just about the finance. "Caring is the essence of nursing; and, unfortunately, caring behaviors may not be easily visible in a health care today. The practice framework, Relationship Based Care, provides an avenue to promote a caring environment"[10] supporting this core essence of nursing. The culture change resulting from the implementation of professional practice model strengthens the team and the care provided. The suggested grassroots approach facilitates change from within the individual units and provides a way forward to achieve lasting culture change.

EXPLANATION OF HCAHPS

The HCAHPS survey is a national, standardized survey that assesses adult patients' perceptions of their hospital stay.[14] It was developed by CMS and the Agency for Healthcare Research and Quality in 2005. The goal of HCAHPS is to provide an objective comparison tool for hospital consumers, incentivize hospitals to improve the quality of care, and enhance accountability in health care. The survey assesses items such as communication with nurses and physicians, pain management, responsiveness of hospital staff, explanations about medications, discharge information, the hospital environment, and overall hospital ratings. Administration of the survey to a random sampling of adult patients began in October 2006 and the first results were posted on the Hospital Compare Web site in March of 2008. There are specific rules regarding inclusion and exclusion criteria. Patients 18 years and older that have had at least an overnight hospital stay, do not have a primary psychiatric diagnosis, and are alive at discharge are some of the inclusion criteria. Patients excluded are prisoners, patients with a foreign address, and "not-for-publication" patients. Patients are also excluded if they are discharged into hospice care, to a skilled nursing facility, or to a nursing home.[15]

REFERENCES

1. Centers for Medicare & Medicaid Services. Frequently asked questions hospital value-based purchasing program. 2012. Available at: https://www.cms.gov/Hospital-Value-BasedPurchasing/Downloads/HVBPFAQ030812.pdf. Accessed March 8, 2012.
2. Shoemaker P. What value-based purchasing means to your hospital. Healthc Financ Manage 2011;65(8):60–8.
3. Professional Research Consultants. (n.d.) HCAHPS VBP calculator for PRCEasyView.com® dimensions for concentration. Available at: https://www.prceasyview.com. Accessed October 23, 2011.
4. Hoffart N, Woods C. Elements of a nursing professional practice model. J Prof Nurs 1996;12(6):354–64.
5. Koloroutis M, Manthey M, Felgen J, et al. Relationship-based care: a model for transforming practice. Minneapolis (MN): Creative Health Care Management; 2004.
6. Winsett R, Hauck S. Implementing relationship-based care. J Nurs Adm 2011; 41(6):285–90.
7. Rosser M. Making relationship-based care a reality. Health Prog 2008;89(3):74–5.
8. Watson J. Caring theory as an ethical guide to administrative and clinical practices. This article is being reprinted with permission from nursing administration quarterly 2006;30(1):48–55. JONAS Healthc Law Ethics Regul 2006;8(3):87–93.
9. Swanson KM. Empirical development of a middle range theory of caring. Nurse Res 1991;40(3):161–6.
10. Mathes S. Implementing a caring model. Creat Nurs 2011;17(1):36–42.
11. Noble DJ, Lemer C, Stanton E. What has change management in industry got to do with improving patient safety? Postgrad Med J 2011;87(1027):345–8. http://dx.doi.org/10.1136/pgmj.2010.097923.
12. Kotter International. The 8-step process for leading change. 2011. Available at: http://kotterinternational.com/kotterprinciples/changesteps. Accessed November 20, 2011.
13. Dingman SK, Williams M, Fosbinder D, et al. Implementing a caring model to improve patient satisfaction. J Nurs Adm 1999;29(12):30–7.
14. Centers for Medicare & Medicaid Services. HCAHPS fact sheet updated. 2010. Available at: http://www.hcahpsonline.org/home.aspx. Accessed October 23, 2011.
15. Centers for Medicare & Medicaid Services. HCAHPS Update Training [PowerPoint slides]. 2011. Available at: http://www.hcahpsonline.org/trainingmaterials.aspx. Accessed October 2, 2011.

A Nursing Leadership and Practice Framework for Success in the Era of Transparency

Patricia A. Cornett, EdD, MS, RN[a,b,*]

KEYWORDS

- Positional leadership • Leadership practice framework • Optimizing microsystems

KEY POINTS

- Rules of continuous healing relationships; patient-controlled, customized, and safe care in which their needs are anticipated; knowledge sharing; and clinician cooperation can only be fully developed, implemented, and sustained when environments created by middle managers facilitate such processes.
- Positional leaders in the twenty-first century, particularly those leading microsystems, must optimize each microsystem through a leadership framework that integrates a focus on people with an evidence-based approach.
- The interplay of the 5 functions in the Positional Leadership Framework is a unifying road map for optimizing clinical microsystems' performance.

Twelve years ago, the Institute of Medicine (IOM) launched a series of studies on the American health care delivery system with its first report, *To Err Is Human; Building a Safer Healthcare System*,[1] in which the extent of medical errors in the American health system were identified. The following year, the second report, *Crossing the Quality Chasm; a New Health System for the 21st Century*,[2] introduced a new framework for improving broken systems of care that included 6 core values of what health care should be: safe, effective, patient-centered, timely, efficient, and equitable. The report further explicated 10 simple rules (**Table 1**) for a redesigned system of delivery of care.

To effect the dramatic changes necessary to implement the 10 simple rules called for changes in organizations' culture, structures, and processes along with change in health professionals' norms and ethics. The report aptly described that, "The current system shows too little cooperation and teamwork. Instead, each discipline

[a] Solúcion Associates, LCC, Canyon Lake, TX, USA; [b] Graduate Administration Program, School of Nursing, The University of Texas Health Science Center at San Antonio, San Antonio, TX, USA
* Corresponding author. 8201 South Santa Fe Drive #255, Littleton, CO 80120.
E-mail address: solucionassociates@gmail.com

Perioperative Nursing Clinics 7 (2012) 305–313
http://dx.doi.org/10.1016/j.cpen.2012.06.001
1556-7931/12/$ – see front matter © 2012 Elsevier Inc. All rights reserved.

Table 1	
Simple rules for the twenty-first century health care system	
Prereport Approach	**New Rule**
Episodic face-to-face clinician-patient visits	1. Care is based on continuous healing relationships
Minimal customization	2. Care is customized according to patient needs and values
Professionals control information that is maintained in closed-record systems	3. The patient is the source of control 4. Knowledge is shared and information flows freely
Variability occurs based on location and clinician	5. Decision making is evidence based
To do no harm is an individual professional responsibility	6. Safety is a system property
Service availability and outcome information are difficult to access	7. Transparency is necessary
System reacts to events	8. Patient needs are anticipated
Efficiency is a high priority	9. Waste is continuously decreased
Professional silos dominate	10. Cooperation among clinicians is a priority

Data from Institute of Medicine. Crossing the quality chasm: a new health system for the 21st century. Washington, DC: National Academies Press; 2001. p. 8–9.

and type of organization tends to defend its authority at the expense of the total system's function—a problem known as suboptimization. Under the new rules, cooperation in patient care is more important than professional prerogatives and roles."[2(p83)] In twenty-first century health care, practitioners' effectiveness is more closely tied to the characteristics of the systems in which they practice. "Quality health care cannot be delivered through a cottage industry any longer. Healthcare today is more and more an interaction between the system and a person who needs help from that system."[2(p6)] The report further stated the purpose of the health care system is to reduce the burden of illness, injury, and disability and to improve the health status and function of the people of the United States.[2] Of all the new rules, transparency has become a particularly important requirement. It is important to first understand what is meant by transparency in health care.

The IOM defined transparency in this context as a health care system that makes information available to patients and their families so they may make informed decisions when selecting a health plan, hospital or clinical practice, or choosing among alternative treatments. Information describing a system's performance on safety, evidence-based practice, and patient satisfaction should be included.[2] That definition has been operationalized in 2 subsets: (1) price transparency for services and products provided by all health care stakeholders to patients, and (2) performance transparency for services and products provided to patients. The often-heard phrase, the era of transparency, seems to mean the age of accessibility to information on a health care system's quality, efficiency, and patient experiences with care received. Despite the abundance of data available today on the Web, only 7% of survey participants in the Kaiser Family Foundation 2008 survey said that they had seen and used information comparing the quality of hospitals to make health care decisions in the prior year, and only 6% said that they had seen and used information comparing physicians.[3] A recent study by Ryan and colleagues[4] concluded that there is little evidence suggesting that consumers use online information to make more informed choices about where to check in for an elective procedure. Levy[5] purports that "transparency's major societal and strategic imperative is to provide creative tension within hospitals so they hold themselves accountable. This accountability is what will drive doctors, nurses, and administrators to seek constant improvements in the quality and safety of patient care." The concept of creative tension originated with Peter Senge,[6] who wrote that "Creative tension comes from seeing clearly where we want to be, our vision, and telling the truth about where we are, our current reality. The gap between the two generates a natural tension." Addressing that gap stimulates creative energy in people and teams from which solutions emerge. There is direct applicability of using creative tension and actualizing the other 9 rules to the formal role of nurse leaders in all care settings.

The focus of this article is on a framework for leader practice that outlines the structure and process for leaders in complex adaptive systems such as health care, in which multilevels of systems exist: microsystem, mesosystem, and macrosystem. Direct care is delivered in a microsystem, such as a postanesthesia unit, outpatient clinic, intervention center, or procedural area such as an operating room, and is supported by the mesosystem and macrosystem levels. To achieve the IOM's call to provide quality care (microsystem level), midlevel leaders (mesosystem) must focus on each microsystem in which the direct care or service is produced.[2] The systems framework depicted in **Fig. 1** informs the functions of the mesosystem to support and develop each microsystem in which patient care is delivered.

Leaders in every industry are the key drivers for creation of quality work environments. Nurse leaders at the mesosystem level are key drivers for creation of work environments in which quality patient care outcomes consistently occur at the microsystem level, which is the front line of health care delivery. Their charge is provision of leadership to ensure quality nursing care, and ensure satisfaction of all stakeholders (patients, families, staff, physicians, and hospital executives) at every clinical care site within their span of control. With the high proportion of professionals in health care, it is essential that nurse leaders actively share leadership through inclusion. There are numerous internal and external interactions and relationships that influence

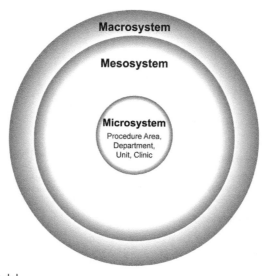

Fig. 1. Systems model.

the dynamic day-to-day functioning of microsystems and it is those professionals in the microsystems who can and do influence processes and outcomes.

The outcome expected of twenty-first century health care leaders at the mesosystem level is to create a health care system that is responsive to those persons who need help from that system. As stewards of that purpose, the task is to build the most important equity, human capital, by encouraging the staff to work collaboratively and cooperatively. The goal is "to help form an environment in which people hold them themselves accountable to the standard of performance that reflects and reinforces the purpose of the company."[7(p3)] The nature of that task and goal and how they can be accomplished are depicted in **Fig. 2**. It is a mental model for understanding the work; a framework for the practice of positional leadership in health care today.

An organization cannot succeed without position leadership. South American poet Antonio Machado[8] declared "... your footsteps are the road...there is no road, the road is made by walking." For the individual in a leadership role, the Positional Leadership Framework guides the footsteps and creates the road to stewardship.

ANALYZE

There are 5 functional categories in the model. Analyze is the central function because, without structured and disciplined analysis, the road map for the other 4 categories fades and is equivalent to wandering in the wilderness without a compass. The Analyze process is essentially the intelligence cycle used in multiple industries for decades.[9] The first step in Analyze is the collection of data. This can entail formal, systematic collection of quantitative or qualitative data, or a collection of seemingly

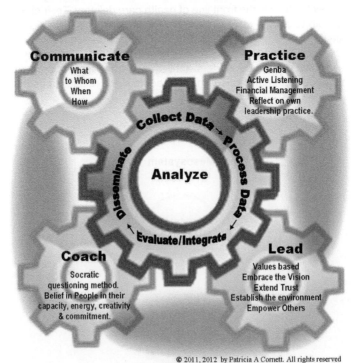

Fig. 2. Cornett framework for positional leadership.

unconnected information. The next step is to process the data, during which it is converted from raw information to a readily useable form of standardized formats such as percentages or percentiles, or for qualitative data, categorized under major themes or organizational performance pillars. The third step is evaluation and integration, during which data are interpreted, correlated, and analyzed in context to ensure credibility and applicability. This step transforms data from mere information to organizational intelligence. For example, viewing data on monthly operating room (OR) scheduled cases and start times is merely review of OR schedule information. Review of a trend report, benchmarked against predetermined goals with categorical subscale analysis by procedure, surgeon, or day of week, is review of intelligence data. Another example is surgeon complaints. Reviewing complaints as isolated incidents and acting on them as such is acting on information as opposed to processing, evaluating, and integrating the data to determine whether trends or themes emerge related to specific surgeons, equipment manufacturers, assigned staff, or other elements.

The final step is dissemination, which is linked to the larger Communicate function. What should be disseminated to whom; at what time, place, or committee meeting; and how it should be disseminated (verbally, written report, before briefing) are all considerations depending on the nature of the product of the analysis.

LEAD

Lead and Coach are the foundational gears of positional leadership. Both highly influence the other 2 functions of Practice and Communicate. Leading must be values based: it must be authentic and ethical. An authentic and ethical leader is a person who has a positive moral perspective, promotes a positive psychological and ethical climate, openly shares information and expressions of own thoughts and feelings, encourages diverse viewpoints, objectively analyzes data before coming to a decision, builds collaborative relationships with followers, has a passion for and commitment to the purpose of the organization, and extends trust throughout the organization.[10,11]

The existence or lack of trust has a direct impact according to Covey.[12] He states:

Trust impacts us 24/7, 365 days a year. It undergirds and affects the quality of every relationship, every communication, every work project, every business venture, every effort in which we are engaged. It changes the quality of every present moment and alters the trajectory and outcome of every future moment of our lives – both personally and professionally.[12(p27)]

According to Covey,[12] there are 12 behaviors that establish subordinates' trust of the leader: listen first, talk straight, show loyalty, show respect and concern, clarify expectations, practice accountability, keep commitments, create transparency, confront reality, right wrongs, get better, and deliver. Leaders' consistent practice of these trust-building behaviors enables trust to be extended throughout an organization as others adopt the same behaviors.[13] Levy[7] attributes his effectiveness as a leader in several different industries to his trust in subordinates. The underlying tenet is belief that subordinates share values that are in consonance with the business purpose of the organization.

Establishing structural and psychological empowerment are the underpinnings of a healthy work environment. According to Kanter,[13] structural empowerment occurs when employees are given opportunity, information, and autonomy; power over their work conditions. In addition, their access to information and leader support and provision of resources results in higher levels of self-efficacy, higher levels of job satisfaction, and increased organization commitment.[13]

In her multidimensional measure of psychological empowerment, Spreitzer[14] explains that psychological empowerment is achieved when staff members have autonomy to influence the outcomes of their work, confidence in their skills to do the work, and when the meaningfulness of their work is promoted. Thus, to create an environment in which staff can excel, leaders should focus on being transparent with information to enable a state of creative tension (the gap between actual and desired state) whereby opportunity for staff to design the solutions manifests itself to collapse the gap and bring increased meaningfulness to their work.

COACH

Effective coaches trust and respect their players. Coaches believe in their players and think that players' innate love of the game and desire to win can be harnessed to create a team that has the collective ability to succeed.[7] Professionals and support personnel in health care choose their work because they want to cure or care for others; they want to make a difference. Belief in their energy, creativity, commitment, and capacity to keep changing to find what works is what keeps the organization alive. Coaching such talented people is about engaging in dialogue through thoughtful and respectful questioning to elicit their understanding and ideas, and show genuine interest in their thinking and decision making. To coach is to make the most of the organization's most valuable resources: the people.

COMMUNICATE

Accurate, timely communication between practitioners is basic to provision of safe patient care. First identified in the IOM report *To Err is Human*[1] as a major factor in medication errors, communication continues to be a major element in success or failure within macrosystem, mesosystem, and microsystem levels. To address the patient safety hazard related to communication, health care borrowed a hand-off briefing technique used in nuclear submarines, then standardized and disseminated it, now known as ISBAR (introduction, situation, background, assessment, recommendation). Standardizing the structure and process of information exchange between clinicians has significantly decreased error rates.[15]

Real-time dissemination of the What, to Whom, When, and How aspects of communication has improved in other ways over the past decade because of millions of hours and dollars spent on standardizing and digitizing health care information, along with e-mail, cell phones, texting, blogging, tweeting, YouTube, and Facebook. Collaboration of clinicians and the sharing of knowledge and information has, and is, occurring.

No matter what communication medium is used, how you say something matters, particularly for leaders whose every word carries influence and meaning. Therapeutic communication that emphasizes listening, respect, talking honestly, and 2-way dialogue establishes a positive mindset. In health care, the primary intent of most communication between clinicians is exchange of information about patients. Information relayed in a nontherapeutic way puts the patient at risk because the receiver of the communication hears and reacts to the disrespect rather than the substantive content of the message. The same holds true for exchange of information between leaders about structure and processes and between leaders and followers. Nontherapeutic communication places the organization at risk when solutions and resolutions are delayed because of interpersonal acrimony.

For those seeking to improve communication skills, a plethora of workshops, e-learning, and books are readily available. Google the phrase "crucial or critical conversation" and more than 50 million resources are cited in less than 12 seconds.

PRACTICE

Practice in the Positional Leadership Framework is the hands-on activity. What is Genba? (The Japanese word *Genba* is sometimes spelled *Gemba*, which is the romanticized version. Either spelling has the same meaning. The words are used interchangeably in the English language literature.) The Japanese Toyota production process, known to many as the Lean process, promotes the 3 Gs: *Genba* (the place where value is created), *Genbutsu* (the thing that is created), and *Genjitsu* (the situation or environment).[16] The philosophy behind the 3 Gs is that, when there is a problem, one should get as close to it as possible before proposing a solution. This approach is also known as Management by Walking Around (MBWA), popularized by the founders of Hewlett Packard, and, later, Tom Peters declared that it was the foundation for leadership and excellence in his second book *A Passion for Excellence: The Leadership Difference*.[17]

The best practice for the health care mesosystem leader is to go to Genba, or round in the microsystem; the department, unit, or procedural areas where value is created. This activity is not aimless, nor is the objective to check on compliance with policies, procedures, or customer service scripts. The purpose is threefold: (1) to listen to what those on the front line are saying; (2) to ask questions, to elicit their ideas; and (3) to experience their situation. Interaction with microsystem-level clinicians occurs at *Genba*, in which leader active listening is paramount.

The concept of reflective practice was first introduced by Dewey[18] in 1933, followed by Argyris[19] and then Schön.[20] It is a defining characteristic of professional practice according to Schön that reflection on one's actions is engagement in continuous learning and improvement of self. Reflection is an essential behavior for the leader to look within and validate that one's leading, coaching, and communicating behaviors are authentic and ethical.

The classic budget and financial responsibilities inherent in any positional leadership role are an integral part of practice. Competence in such is expected, but not in lieu of competence in the other areas of leadership practice.

What leaders learned in the past about leading is no longer adequate in today's chaotic, complex health care environment. It is essential to engage others and capitalize on the untapped intuition and insights of frontline staff. In **Fig. 3**, the Positional

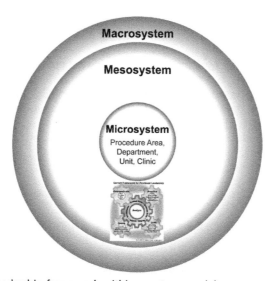

Fig. 3. Position leadership framework within a systems model.

Leadership Framework has been embedded in the systems model to depict actualization of leader behaviors and actions at the mesosystem level to facilitate the work of those concentrated in microsystems of the organization.

SUMMARY

The 10 supposedly simple rules put forth by the IOM are not simple in concept or in implementation. Those rules of continuous healing relationships; patient-controlled, customized, and safe care in which their needs are anticipated; knowledge sharing; and clinician cooperation can only be fully developed, implemented, and sustained when environments created by middle managers facilitate such processes. Positional leaders in the twenty-first century, particularly those leading microsystems, must optimize each microsystem through a leadership framework that integrates a focus on people with an evidence-based approach. The interplay of the 5 functions in the Positional Leadership Framework is a unifying road map for optimizing the performance of clinical microsystems.

REFERENCES

1. Institute of Medicine. To err is human: building a safer healthcare system. Washington, DC: National Academies Press; 2000.
2. Institute of Medicine. Crossing the quality chasm: a new health system for the 21st century. Washington, DC: National Academies Press; 2001.
3. Lindenauer P. Public reporting and pay-for-performance programs in perioperative medicine. Are they meeting their goals? Cleve Clin J Med 2009;76(S4):53–8. Available at: http://www.ccjm.org/content/76/Suppl_4/S3.full.pdf+html. Accessed April 2, 2012.
4. Ryan A, Nallamothu B, Dimick J. Medicare's public reporting initiative on hospital quality had modest or no impact on mortality from three key conditions. Health Aff 2012;31(3):585–92.
5. Levy P. Speech at MIT Club of Northern California. Berkeley (CA); 2010. Available at: http://vimeo.com/10082781. Accessed March 16, 2012.
6. Senge P. The leaders new work. Society for Organizational Learning. Available at: http://www.solonline.org/res/kr/newwork.html. Accessed March 12, 2012.
7. Levy P. Goal play. Lexington (KY): Createspace; 2012.
8. Machado A. Available at: http://www.goodreads.com/quotes/show/8837. Accessed March 15, 2012.
9. The intelligence cycle. Available at: www.dtic.mil/doctrine/jrm/intl4.ppt. Accessed March 15, 2012.
10. Bennis W. The essence of leadership. National Technological University Corporation and Linkage, Inc; 1999. Available at: http://www.ntu.edu/notes/BusManChannel/notes/TNEL0000_pm.pdf. Accessed February 21, 2012.
11. Walumbwa F, Avolio B, Gardner W, et al. Authentic leadership: development and validation of a theory-based measure. J Manag 2008;34(1):89–126.
12. Covey SM. The speed of trust. The one thing that changes everything. New York: Free Press; 2006.
13. Kanter R. Men and women of the corporation. 2nd edition. New York: Basic Books; 1993.
14. Spreitzer G. Social, structural characteristics of psychological empowerment. Acad Manage J 1996;39(2):483–504.
15. Haig K, Sutton S, Whittington J. SBAR: a shared mental model for improving communication between clinicians. Jt Comm J Qual Patient Saf 2006;32(31): 167–75.

16. From: Training with Industry. Available at: http://trainingwithinindustry.blogspot. com/2008/12/genba-genbutsu-genjitsu-in-plain.html. Accessed March 31, 2012.
17. Peters T, Austin N. A passion for excellence: the leadership difference. New York: Grand Central Publishing; 1985.
18. Dewey J. How we think. A restatement of the relation of reflective thinking to the educative process. Revised edition. Boston: DC Heath; 1933.
19. Argyris C, Schön D. Organization learning: a theory of action perspective. Reading (MA): Addison-Wesley; 1978.
20. Schön D. The reflective practitioner, how professionals think in action. New York: Basic Books; 1983.

Evaluating an Innovative Educational Strategy for Health Care Organizations

Building Bridges Across Historical Silos for Quality

Andrea E. Berndt, PhD[a],*, Mickey Parsons, PhD, MSN, RN[b],
Clarice Golightly-Jenkins, PhD, MSN, RN, CNS[c]

KEYWORDS

- Collaboration • Innovation • Interprofessional learning
- Learning practice communities • Quality improvement

KEY POINTS

- As learning practice communities take hold in hospitals, interdisciplinary learning will become the norm as opposed to the exception and facilitate the transformation needed in delivery of patient care.
- In an effort to create a learning practice community and enhance the success of quality-improvement (QI) initiatives at a large urban hospital system, plans were made to develop and implement an interprofessional quality study group to facilitate shared goals between nurse educators and quality directors.
- Development of these interprofessional partnerships was viewed as essential to guide and promote QI goals at the facility level with nurse coordinators and their staff.

The current health care environment has created an imperative for collaboration between hospitals' nurse educators, quality directors, physicians, and clinical nurse leaders at the macrosystem and microsystem levels. Collaboration requires open communication between professionals from differing disciplines, settings, and

Disclosure statement: None of the authors has financial relationships with commercial companies that have direct financial relationships to the subject matter in this article.
Note: There are no drug or equipment trademarks appearing in this article.
[a] School of Nursing, The University of Texas Health Science Center at San Antonio, Family and Community Health Systems Department, 7703 Floyd Curl Drive, MC 7950, San Antonio, TX 78229, USA; [b] The University of Texas Health Science Center at San Antonio, School of Nursing, Health Care Restoration and Systems Management, 7703 Floyd Curl Drive, MC 7975, San Antonio, TX 78229, USA; [c] Methodist Healthcare System, John E. Hornbeak Building, 4450 Medical Drive Suite 3112, San Antonio, TX 78229, USA
* Corresponding author.
E-mail address: Berndt@uthscsa.edu

degrees of power to develop innovative solutions for change based on shared outcomes.[1–5] Collaboration and communication, however, cannot be assumed merely because various health care professionals are sitting and talking in the same room.

The training of health care professionals differs in terms of their conceptual frameworks, research methods, and terminology, which can impede their ability to promote translational research across their disciplines.[6–8] As noted in the recent Institute of Medicine report on the *The Future of Nursing*,[9] however, collaboration between organizational leaders and health care practitioners is a key strength to ensure the innovation needed for quality in patient care.

Moreover, many hospitals have rigid organizational structures and disciplinary silos that serve to perpetuate cultural divides and communication difficulties.[4,10,11] One way to break down these barriers is by forming learning practice communities in which interdependent health care professionals work together toward shared goals and, in so doing, create new collective identities that help them achieve those goals.

These new collective identities, learning practice communities, exist when individuals with a shared vision and goals create a transformative learning environment.[12–16] The success of these communities is greater than that of traditional learning experiences due to several important distinctions. First, there is an emphasis on creating a culture of collective rather than individual learning. Second, a learning practice community works to develop and maintain systematic, continuous learning routines. Third, a learning practice community builds in time for reflection, adaptations, modifications, and skill development. Finally, because learning practice communities base interactions and communication on mutual respect and trust, those participating are more often fully engaged in the process. Such engagement increases the likelihood that members question assumptions and see the limitations in trying to solve problems rather than prevent them. Furthermore, this engagement promotes openness and a willingness to embrace opportunities revealed in new approaches, ideas, and viewpoints.

As learning practice communities take hold in hospitals, interdisciplinary learning will become the norm as opposed to the exception and facilitate the transformation needed in delivery of patient care. By breaking down existing silos that encourage isolated decisions and combining the skills and insights of administrators and bedside clinicians, the success of QI initiatives focused on patient-centered care will increase.

In an effort to create a learning practice community and enhance the success of QI initiatives at a large urban hospital system, plans were made to develop and implement an interprofessional quality study group (ISG) to facilitate shared goals between nurse educators and quality directors. Development of these interprofessional partnerships was viewed as essential to guide and promote QI goals at the facility level with nurse coordinators and their staff. To enhance the quality of these partnerships, several outcomes were identified: (1) provide a common language and background across facilities and individuals, (2) increase knowledge of QI measurement approaches and learn how to use available data for meaningful application, (3) plan QI initiatives proactively, and (4) help point-of-care staff connect the dots and engender ownership of QI initiatives.

METHOD
Participants

A formal invitation to participate in the Interprofessional Study Group for Quality Improvement (ISG) was sent to nursing educators and quality directors (N = 20) at each of the hospital's 8 primary facilities from the hospital's vice president for education and research. The decision to invite participants, rather than require attendance, was intentional, because prior research indicated that accepting an invitation to learn leads to greater engagement in the process.[17] Given the number of invitations sent, no more than 20 individuals were expected to attend the first sessionand fewer to commit to the full process.

The Conceptual Framework

The ISG was designed around several principles: (1) to create a learning practice community, (2) to break down existing silos via interprofessional learning, and (3) to provide a common language and knowledge of QI design and measurement to meet the IOM's 6 aims for twenty-first century health care systems.[18]

In keeping with the themes of interprofessional learning and learning practice communities, the developers of the ISG included the hospital's chief quality officer, the vice president for quality management and clinical outcomes, the vice president for education and research, and 2 professors from a nearby university school of nursing. Before the start of the ISG, a logic model was developed and presented to the hospital's vice president for education and research and to the chief quality officer for review. The ISG objectives, outcomes, outcome indicators, and assessment instruments are listed in **Table 1**.

Design and Delivery of ISG Sessions

To increase the likelihood of regular attendance, all 13 ISG sessions were scheduled at approximately noon and limited to a maximum of 90 minutes. All sessions occurred between October 1, 2011, and February 29, 2012. Gourmet catered meals were available at the beginning of each session, providing participants with an additional benefit and further demonstrating the health systems' commitment to the endeavor. Beyond

Table 1
Objectives, outcomes, and outcome indicators for the Interprofessional Study Group for Quality Improvement

Objectives	Discuss *Value by Design* content from the Dartmouth QI curriculum.
	Enhance discussion of *Value by Design* content using facilitated discussion methodology.
	Collaborate, communicate, and solve problems related to quality/patient safety issues.
	Apply the Dartmouth QI approach and tools to improve patient care at their facility.
	Identify and select different measurement approaches to measure specific outcomes.
Outcomes	Interview a patient to increase awareness and understanding of health care experiences.
	Identify a priority quality gap from patient interviews and facility level data.
	Propose a pilot QI initiative based on the identified quality gap
	Present the proposed QI initiative to all ISG participants.
	Indicators
	PowerPoint presentations, verbal summaries, and written handouts.
	Increase readiness for interprofessional learning.
	Indicators
	Baseline and post-test scores on RIPLS.
	Open-ended comments from the post-test evaluation questions.
	Create an interprofessional learning practice community.
	Indicators
	Baseline and post-test scores on the LPI.
	Open-ended comments from the post-test evaluation questions.

weekly meals, participants also received 2 books—*Value by Design*,[19] from The Dartmouth Institute's QI curriculum, and *William Fawcett Hill's Learning Through Discussion.*[20]

At the first ISG session, all attendees came to consensus on rules for engagement during each session and identified outcomes to attain by the end of the sessions. In addition, the first session was used to administer baseline outcome indicators. To create interprofessional learning practice communities and ensure that learning was relevant and meaningful, participants were grouped by their facility to serve as book chapter facilitators and patient interview teams. These groupings resulted in 8 teams and reflected the full diversity of the health system's primary facilities.

For 9 of the 13 sessions, the first 60 minutes were devoted to discussion and facilitation of chapter content from *Value by Design*,[19] and the final 30 minutes were set aside to discuss upcoming plans, answer questions and/or address conflicts, discuss patient interviews, or review progress toward pilot projects. The facilitation structure for the first 60 minutes was constant across sessions and delivered in the following sequence: (1) check-in, (2) review of chapter vocabulary, (3) identify the chapter's general statement and major themes, (4) apply chapter material to other areas and self, and (5) evaluate the presentation of the chapter and the facilitating team's discussion of the content. The methodology and facilitation structure was based on the group discussion guide, *William Fawcett Hill's Learning Through Discussion.*[20]

Of the remaining 4 sessions, 1 was set aside for participants to summarize the content of their patient interviews, and 2 were reserved for participants to present their proposed QI initiatives. Post-test administration of the outcome indicators took place after presentations at the final session.

Assessment Instruments

The Readiness for Interprofessional Learning Scale (RIPLS)[21–24] was developed to assess students' readiness for interprofessional learning and is composed of 3 subscales: teamwork and collaboration, professional identity, and roles and responsibilities. This 19-item scale uses a 5-point Likert scale ranging from 1 (strongly disagree) to 5 (strongly agree). The scale has been used primarily with students from many health care disciplines (eg, dentistry, medicine, nursing, and pharmacy).[22,24] Reliability for recent versions of the RIPLS has ranged from 0.70 to 0.88.

In addition, the RIPLS was extended to 29 items in 2004 to strengthen items assessing roles and responsibilities and evaluate new items assessing patient centeredness. A 2006 study in Scotland administered this 29-item RIPLS and compared responses between 66 general practitioners, 210 nurses, 45 pharmacists, and 223 allied health professionals.[23] The results supported 2 of the original subscales (teamwork and collaboration and professional identity) and 1 new subscale (patient centeredness). Their results, however, could not support 1 original subscale (roles and responsibilities). Moreover, these investigators noted differences in subscale responses as a function of professional status. Specifically, nurses and allied health professionals had significantly higher scores on teamwork and collaboration and patient centeredness and significantly lower scores on professional identity. Although these results are intriguing, no other studies seem to have used this extended scale. Thus, for the current evaluation, 1 of the original 19 items was removed due to its specific focus on classroom education, and the remaining items were modified by replacing the term, *student*, with the term, *health care professional*.

The Learning Practice Inventory (LPI) was developed for primary care practices in the United Kingdom by Rushmer and colleagues.[13,16] The original LPI has 62 items and assesses the extent to which 3 domains of learning practice communities (engagement, learning, and support) are perceived to exist in the health care setting. **Table 2**

Table 2
Learning Practice Inventory domains and definitions

LPI Domain	Definition
Engagement (14 items)	The extent to which health professionals exhibit ownership, involvement, supportive attitudes, and beliefs that collective learning was safe and expected in the organization
Learning (20 items)	The extent to which health professionals develop and persist in collective learning routines to share and search for knowledge, clinical expertise, and problem solving, resulting in process improvements and positive outcomes
Support (20 items)	The extent to which organizational resources, education and training, and information and information systems support health professionals' behaviors to learn collectively

presents the definitions for the 3 LPI domains. In 2 recent studies, reliability for the LPI subscales ranged from 0.73 to 0.94.[15] For this study, the original LPI was reduced from 62 to 55 items to ease participant burden, and the wording for items was modified as needed to facilitate understanding for participants in the United States.

Finally, at the post-test, an open-ended evaluation form with 2 questions was used to solicit participant feedback about their experience in the ISG. The first question asked participants to report their greatest insight or take-away idea from the experience. The second question asked participants to report what they liked most and least about the experience.

RESULTS
Participants

At the first session, there were 11 directors of nursing education and 10 quality directors in attendance (N = 21). The total number of participants at the final session was 18 (11 directors of nursing education and 7 quality directors). At baseline and post-test, 2 noticeable differences were evident between the groups (**Table 3**). First, although more than half of the nursing educators reported prior experiences with interprofessional learning, only 1 quality director indicated a prior interprofessional learning experience. Second, the quality directors exhibited greater variation in length of time at their facility and in their role.

Table 4 presents baseline and post-test means and standard deviations for the RIPLS and LPI subscale scores. Inspection of baseline and post-test scores for the RIPLS yielded evidence that participants were moderately positive about professional

Table 3
Baseline and post-test characteristics of directors of nursing education and quality directors

	Characteristic	Range	Baseline (N = 11) Mean (SD)	Post-Test (N = 11) Mean (SD)
Nursing education directors	Time in the facility	17–144	64.92 (46.40)	70.73 (43.89)
	Time in the role	7–244	45.25 (31.12)	49.27 (34.65)
			Baseline (N = 10) Mean (SD)	Post-Test (N = 7) Mean (SD)
Quality directors	Time in the facility	2–288	83.80 (74.70)	106.86 (95.75)
	Time in the role	5–130	63.30 (46.41)	59.10 (43.70)

Time in the facility and role is expressed in number of months.

Table 4
Baseline and post-test means and standard deviations for the LPI and RIPLS

Assessment Instrument	Subdomains	Range	Pre-Test Mean (SD)	Post-Test Mean (SD)
LPI	Engagement	14–126	100.1 (16.6)	103.1 (16.9)
	Learning	20–180	122.1 (31.9)	126.3 (30.7)
	Support	20–180	122.9 (28.6)	130.7 (25.1)
RIPLS	Professional identity	8–40	34.0 (7.66)	33.6 (4.63)
	Roles/responsibilities	1–5	2.8 (1.25)	2.9 (1.21)
	Teamwork/collaboration	9–45	39.6 (8.46)	42.2 (3.75)

identity and extremely positive about teamwork and collaboration. In contrast, baseline and post-test scores for roles and responsibilities were less positive. On 2 RIPLS subscales (professional identity and roles and responsibilities), scores were stable from baseline to post-test. Scores for teamwork and collaboration were slightly higher at post-test than at baseline and demonstrated greater consistency.

Similarly, inspection of baseline and post-test scores for all LPI subscales indicated substantial stability in responses. Of the 3 subscales, participants were most positive about the degree to which characteristics of engagement were present in their work setting. Perceptions about the degree to which characteristics of learning and support were present were also positive but less positive than perceptions regarding the presence of engagement characteristics.

To examine if there was a difference between participants' RIPLS or LPI subscale responses from baseline to post-test, dependent t tests were performed. Given the stability in subscale mean scores of both instruments, the total lack of differences was not surprising. Moreover, no differences were evident when baseline and post-test scores were compared between directors of nursing education and quality directors.

Although there were no differences in the subscale scores of the RIPLS and the LPI, it was also of interest to determine if there were any changes to individual items from the RIPLS or the LPI. Given the small sample size, a probability level of .10 was used for significance. Interpretation from a series of dependent t tests revealed significant increases on 1 RIPLS item and on 7 items from the LPI (see detailed t test information in **Table 5**). A significant decrease was revealed on 1 LPI item. Of the 8 items with differences on the LPI, 1 was from the engagement domain, 1 was from the support domain, and the remaining 6 were from the learning domain.

To examine if relationships existed between baseline and post-test subscale responses from the RIPLS and the LPI, bivariate Pearson correlations were performed. Interpretation of correlation coefficients revealed significant, strong, positive relationships between baseline subscale scores on the RIPLS and all post-test LPI subscales (**Table 6** lists correlation coefficients). Similarly, baseline LPI engagement and learning scores exhibited significant, strong, positive relationships to all post-test LPI subscales. In contrast, baseline scores on the LPI support subscale only evidenced a significant, strong, positive relationship to post-test LPI support scores.

Attitudes and Perceptions

When participants were asked about their main insight or take-away idea from the ISG, there were 3 prominent themes (**Box 1**). First, the majority indicated that they learned the most from one another, hearing different perspectives and seeing different ways to approach their problems. Second, many participants reported that they had

Table 5

Baseline and post-test means and standard deviations for dependent *t* tests (N = 18)

Variable	Mean	SD	Mean Difference	*t* value	*P*
RIPLS: shared learning will help me understand my own professional limitations					
Baseline	4.00	1.24	−0.56	−1.85	.08
Post-test	4.56	0.71			
LPI engagement: I am able to learn new things that are directly relevant to my job					
Baseline	8.22	1.44	−0.50	−1.85	.08
Post-test	8.72	0.46			
LPI support: the organization systematically reviews performance against clearly defined objectives					
Baseline	6.44	2.12	−1.17	−2.58	.02
Post-test	7.61	1.50			
LPI learning: best practices are shared across the organization					
Baseline	6.44	2.06	−0.89	−2.47	.03
Post-test	7.33	1.68			
LPI learning: if the organization has a problem, we find and fix the root cause					
Baseline	5.00	2.66	−1.28	−2.10	.05
Post-test	6.28	2.32			
LPI learning: the organization is committed to educational activities on a regular basis					
Baseline	5.00	2.66	−1.28	−2.10	.06
Post-test	6.28	2.32			
LPI learning: our organization consistently documents if practice changes work well or not					
Baseline	5.33	2.43	−1.22	−2.15	.05
Post-test	6.56	1.38			
LPI learning: our organization delivers a higher quality of health care now than in the past					
Baseline	6.72	1.71	−0.89	−2.05	.06
Post-test	7.61	1.15			
LPI learning: when our organization makes changes, it is after thorough discussion and careful review of benefits and consequences					
Baseline	5.44	2.38	1.44	2.50	.03
Post-test	4.00	1.50			

a new appreciation for quality initiatives, learned important terminology, and identified measurement tools and approaches that they planned to use at their sites. Third, and perhaps most important, participants reported the information gleaned from interviewing patients and their families about their health care experiences provided fresh perspectives from which to view health care delivery in the system. Furthermore, many participants indicated that after completing their patient interviews, they remembered the passion and drive that led them to choose a career in health care.

Discussion and Lessons Learned

To the authors' knowledge, this is one of the first descriptions of an interprofessional learning strategy joining nursing educators and quality directors. The results suggest that participating in the ISG led to more positive attitudes about collaborating with one another, contributed to the development of a common language, and provided greater insights about patients' hospital experiences. These positive reactions may be due to a variety of shared philosophies and goals among the participants.

Table 6
Correlation matrix of pretest and post-test scores for RIPLS and LPI subscales (N = 18)

	Pre-Test RIPLS			Pre-Test LPI			Post-Test RIPLS			Post-Test LPI		
	Profld	Roles	Team	Eng	Lrn	Sup	Profld	Roles	Team	Eng	Lrn	Sup
Pre-test												
RIPLS												
Profld	—											
Roles	0.42	—										
Team	0.83	0.28	—									
LPI												
Eng	0.29	0.08	0.09	—								
Lrn	0.14	0.34	0.17		—							
Sup	0.32	0.23	−0.03			—						
Post-test												
RIPLS												
Profld	−0.06	0.43	−0.13	0.34	0.17	0.36	—					
Roles	−0.05	0.42	−0.32	−0.08	0.22	0.24		—				
Team	0.23	0.06	−0.01	0.39	0.30	0.27			—			
LPI												
Eng	0.66[a]	0.73[a]	0.69[a]	0.66[a]	0.48[b]	0.29	−0.05	−0.35	0.07	—		
Lrn	0.52[b]	0.59[b]	0.55[b]	0.64[a]	0.52[b]	0.37	−0.02	−0.12	0.06		—	
Sup	0.48[b]	0.53[b]	0.43	0.74[a]	0.74[a]	0.59[a]	0.14	−0.26	0.13			—

Abbreviations: Eng, engagement; Lrn, learning; Profld, professional identity; Roles, roles and responsibilities; Sup, support; Team, teamwork and collaboration.
[a] $P<.01$.
[b] $P<.05$.

The organizational culture and context at multiple system levels is a useful lens through which to discuss the process and outcome results. The concept of culture described as existing at the level of visible artifacts, espoused values, and shared tacit assumptions contributes to understanding the context of the system and specific facilities.

During the 4 months that nursing educators and quality directors met for ISG sessions, the organization entered a period of intense uncertainty. These uncertainties, not unusual in the tumultuous world of health care national policy today, have an impact on reimbursement and the financial health of organizations with downstream influence on organizational structure, staffing, and clinical operations. Discussions across the ISG sessions reflected participants' growing concerns about potential changes to the organizational structure. Unfortunately, the administration of post-test outcome indicators occurred when participants' uncertainty about the situation and concern about future decisions seemed to be paramount in their thoughts.

Participants were knowledgeable regarding state and national policy and expressed commitment to becoming life-long learners to lead quality in their roles. Aware of the policy impact, they verbally agreed with the primary goals of the Interprofessional Quality Study Group, which were to (1) to provide a common language and background across facilities and individuals, (2) to increase knowledge of QI measurement approaches and learn how to use available data for meaningful application, (3) to plan QI initiatives proactively, and (4) to help point-of-care staff connect the dots and

---

Box 1

Participant responses to the open-ended post-test questions

Main insight

- Interviewing patients led to eye-opening information
- Better understanding of quality and QI
- The importance of measurement in quality initiatives
- We all have the same end goals

Liked most

- Interviewing and partnering with patients
- Group discussions
- Hearing different perspectives
- Exposure to new tools and information
- Excellent books
- Having opportunities to work as a team
- Enjoyed serving as "teacher" for a book chapter
- Watching teams gel and acting like a "real" team

Liked least

- Carving out time to participate in the study group
- Balancing competing priorities
- Exposure to pre-existing assumptions and negative attitudes
- ISG format led to "overly structured" discussions
- Organizational upheaval and changes in personnel

---

engender ownership of QI initiatives. During the first session, participants indicated that attainment of these goals was an essential strategy to ensure organizational success in the future.

Although the educational program evaluation yielded few significant differences from baseline to post-test, throughout all sessions, participants continued to verbalize their strong commitment to developing a common language and forming a common background to drive quality across the system and within each facility. This qualitative outcome is the strongest result of the educational program. This commitment began the process of establishing a foundation for leadership of interprofessional teams at microsystem levels throughout the system.

Second, the expressed impact and value of the educational strategy of interviewing patients to better understand health care delivery across the system was a key outcome. Given their day-to-day responsibilities, organizational leaders are often removed from patients and families. Participants reported that insights from their patient interviews renewed their commitment to transform health care delivery and reminded them of the passion and caring that led them to their present career.

In keeping with the original objectives proposed for the ISG, participants designed and presented a QI initiative based on their patient interviews and facility-level data. Implementation of these initiatives at the facility level, however, a needed step to help point-of-care staff connect the dots and engender ownership of QI initiatives, could not occur. Given the rapidly changing landscape of the health care system and related environmental uncertainties, the next best step forward was to postpone implementation of QI initiatives until there was less uncertainty in the system. Although this postponement was disappointing to participants, almost all agreed that launching initiatives at a time of upheaval and change was unwise. Therefore, the fourth objective, to move the initiative to the microsystem and point of care, was not achieved.

SUMMARY

Given the report of an expert panel, *Core Competencies for Interprofessional Collaborative Practice*,[25] by nursing, medicine, pharmacy, dentistry, and public health professional education associations, it is essential that current health care providers be prepared for successful interprofessional collaboration for quality care and outcomes. This article has presented an innovative educational program to promote interprofessional collaboration and create a learning practice community. Although there were few significant differences in the quantitative surveys, the participants' verbal feedback provides encouragement that it would be useful to replicate the educational approach with further attention to understanding local organizational culture and context in developing the design.

REFERENCES

1. Bunniss S, Gray F, Kelly D. Collective learning, change and improvement in health care: trialling a facilitated learning initiative with general practice teams. J Eval Clin Pract 2011;18:1–7.
2. Herlehy AM. Influencing safe perioperative practice through collaboration. AORN J 2011;94(3):217–8.
3. Hill KS. Diminishing competition, maximizing benefit through dissemination and collaboration. Nurs Leader 2006;37:24–7.
4. Miller LC, Jones BB, Graves RS, et al. Merging silos: collaborating for information literacy. J Contin Educ Nurs 2010;41(6):267–72.
5. Thannhauser J, Russell-Mayhew S, Scott C. Measures of interprofessional education and collaboration. J Interprof Care 2010;24(4):336–49.
6. Angelini DJ. Interdisciplinary and interprofessional education. J Perinat Neonatal Nurs 2011;25(2):175–9.
7. Lukas CV, Holmes SK, Cohen AB, et al. Transformational change in health care systems: an organizational model. Health Care Manage Rev 2007;32(4):309–20.
8. McNaron ME. Using transformational learning principles to change behavior in the OR. AORN J 2009;89(5):851–60.
9. IOM (Institute of Medicine). The future of nursing: leading change, advancing health. Washington, DC: The National Academies Press; 2011.
10. Margalit R, Thompson S, Visovsky C, et al. From professional silos to interprofessional education: campuswide focus on quality of care. Qual Manag Health Care 2009;18(3):165–73.
11. Newhouse RP, Spring B. Interdisciplinary evidence-based practice: moving from silos to synergy. Nurs Outlook 2010;58:309–17.
12. Herbers MS, Antelo A, Ettling D, et al. Improving teaching through a community of practice. J Transform Educ 2011;9(2):89–108.
13. Rushmer R, Lough M, Wilkinson JE, et al. Introducing the learning practice—I. The characteristics of learning organizations in primary care. J Eval Clin Pract 2004;10(3):375–86.
14. Rushmer R, Kelly D, Lough M, et al. Introducing the learning practice—II. Becoming a learning practice. J Eval Clin Pract 2004;10(3):387–98.

15. Rushmer R, Kelly D, Lough M, et al. Introducing the learning practice—III. Leadership, empowerment, protected time and reflective practice as core contextual conditions. J Eval Clin Pract 2004;10(3):399–405.
16. Rushmer RK, Kelly D, Lough M, et al. The learning practice inventory: diagnosing and developing learning practices in the UK. J Eval Clin Pract 2007;13(2): 206–11.
17. Southern NL. Mentoring for transformative learning: the importance of relationship in creating learning communities of care. J Transform Educ 2007;5(4): 329–38.
18. Institute of Medicine (IOM). Crossing the quality chasm: a new health system for the 21st century. Washington, DC: The National Academies Press; 2001.
19. Nelson E, Batalden P, Godfrey M, et al. Value by design: developing clinical microsystems to achieve organizational excellence. Thousand Oaks (CA): Jossey-Bass; 2011.
20. Rabow J, Charness M, Kipperman J, et al. William Fawcett Hill's learning through discussion. 3rd edition. Long Grove (IL): Waveland Press; 2000.
21. Parsell G, Bligh J. The development of a questionnaire to assess the readiness of health care students for interprofessional learning (RIPLS). Med Educ 1999;33: 95–100.
22. McFayden AK, Webster V, Strachan K, et al. The readiness for Interprofessional learning scale: a possible more stable sub-scale model for the original version of RIPLS. J Interprof Care 2005;19(6):595–603.
23. McFayden AK, Webster VS, Maclaren WM. The test-retest reliability of a revised version of the Readiness for Interprofessional Learning Scale (RIPLS). J Interprof Care 2006;20(6):633–9.
24. Mattick K, Bligh J. An e-resource to coordinate research activity with the Readiness for Interprofessional Learning Scale (RIPLS). J Interprof Care 2005;19(6): 604–13.
25. Interprofessional Education Collaborative Expert Panel. Core competencies for interprofessional collaborative practice. Washington, DC: Interprofessional Education Collaborative; 2011.

Teaching Nurses How to Use Dashboards: A Primer

Gretchel Ajon-Gealogo, MSN, RN-BC, CMSRN

KEYWORDS

- Dashboards • Perioperative nursing • Surgical Care Improvement Project

KEY POINTS

- A Surgical Care Improvement Project (SCIP) primer is a cost-effective and efficient way to disseminate information to frontline nurses whose clinical judgment and practice impact patient care quality and outcomes significantly.
- Dashboards can be powerful visual tools that can help teams highlight opportunities for process and/or performance improvement, celebrate surpassed benchmarks, and set new goals.
- When bringing together the key stakeholders and end users to develop primers and dashboards for the perioperative setting, the real-life problem being addressed is the need for frontline nurses to understand, apply, and disseminate knowledge of SCIP measures.

According to the Centers for Medicare and Medicaid Services (CMS), over $2.5 trillion was spent on health care last year in the United States, roughly 18% of the national gross domestic product.[1] Almost $10 billion has been spent on an excess 2.5 million hospital days resulting from the estimated 750,000 to 1 million surgical site infections reported annually.[2,3] Given these numbers, educating frontline perioperative nurses on understanding and incorporating patient care quality measures into nursing practice must remain a top priority for nursing leaders in academic and clinical settings. In perioperative nursing, patient care standards are outlined in the Surgical Care Improvement Project's (SCIP) evidence-based process measures (**Table 1**), which count among The Joint Commission's (TJC) Core Measures Data Set and were first implemented by the CMS in 2006.[3–5]

Although public disclosure of SCIP data on the Hospital Compare Web site is voluntary, hospitals cannot receive CMS reimbursement without doing so. Furthermore, CMS has instituted a pay-for-performance program that reimburses hospitals based on their ability to meet national benchmarks for these process and outcomes measures.[4]

School of Nursing, The University of Texas Health Science Center San Antonio, 7703 Flyod Curl Drive, San Antonio, TX 78229, USA
E-mail address: gealogo@livemail.uthscsa.edu

Perioperative Nursing Clinics 7 (2012) 327–332
http://dx.doi.org/10.1016/j.cpen.2012.06.004
1556-7931/12/$ – see front matter © 2012 Elsevier Inc. All rights reserved.

Table 1 SCIP core measure set	
SCIP Measure Identifier	Measure Name
SCIP INF-1	Prophylactic antibiotic received within 1 h before surgical incision
SCIP INF-2	Prophylactic antibiotic selection for surgical patients
SCIP INF-3	Prophylactic antibiotics discontinued within 24 h after surgery end time
SCIP INF-4	Cardiac patients with controlled 6 AM postoperative blood glucose
SCIP INF-6	Surgery patients with appropriate hair removal
SCIP INF-9	Urinary catheter removed on postoperative day one (pod 1) or postoperative day two (pod 2) with day of surgery being day zero
SCIP INF-10	Surgery patients with perioperative temperature management
SCIP CARD-2	Surgery patients on beta-blocker therapy before arrival who received a beta-blocker during the perioperative period
SCIP VTE-1	Surgery patients with recommended venous thromboembolism prophylaxis ordered
SCIP VTE-2	Surgery patients who received appropriate venous thromboembolism prophylaxis within 24 h before surgery to 24 h after surgery

Data from QualityNet: National Hospital Quality Measures, Specifications Manual, Discharges 10/01/2009 to 3/31/2010. Available at: www.qualitynet.org. Accessed March 11, 2012.

WHY USE A PRIMER?

SCIP measures and benchmarks are re-evaluated annually and, since their inception, they have evolved with increasing frequency as the evidence base for perioperative practice continues to expand. A primer—that is, a quick reference guide—is a cost-effective and efficient way to disseminate information to frontline nurses whose clinical judgment and practice impact patient care quality and outcomes significantly. A primer specific to perioperative nursing might include a list of the SCIP measures, their definitions, and related local and/or national benchmarks and protocols. Ideally, a primer provides need-to-know information concisely. A card that is portable, durable, and fits nicely in a scrub pocket is suggested. **Fig. 1** is an example of a two-sided SCIP primer card.

Most importantly, a primer should be user-friendly and useful. It should be developed and evaluated by key stakeholders and end users who are committed to reviewing its utility and accuracy on a regular basis. In this way, a primer—and the process undertaken to develop one—may be regarded as a first step in articulating how patient care quality applies to nursing practice. In doing so, a primer can also reinforce that the nurse's responsibility lies beyond completing tasks for a procedure or a shift—it serves as a reminder that nurses are managers of patient outcomes.

WHY USE A DASHBOARD?

A dashboard (also known as storyboard or data wall) is a designated space on which a graphic representation of a clinical microsystem process and outcome-measures data, including present and future benchmarks, is displayed. It may include data on system strengths and/or weaknesses, assets and/or needs, process flowcharts, or action plans. In perioperative nursing, a clinical microsystem might be a surgical team, an inpatient surgery unit, or a postanesthesia care unit. These are all small groups of clinicians, support staff, and patients brought together for a common

SCIP Measures Perioperative Area Checklist	
Prophylactic antibiotic given within 1 hr of surgical incision?	ABX start time: _____ ABX stop time: _____
Prophylactic antibiotic selected?	If selecting non-recommended ABX, reason why:
Appropriate surgical site hair removal?	If removal technique not recommended, reason why:
Perioperative temperature management (required for colorectal surgery)	Post-op normothermia (≥96.8F) within 15 min after leaving OR? ___F If not, time to normothermia: _____
β-blocker therapy prior to arrival?	Med: _____ Last time given: _____
Recommended VTE prophylaxis ordered? _____ If not, reason why: _____	VTE prophylaxis within 24 hrs prior to/after surgery? _____ If not, reason why: _____

Surgical Care Improvement Project (SCIP) Core Measures Data Set	
SCIP INF-1	Prophylactic Antibiotic Received Within 1 Hour Prior to Surgical Incision
SCIP INF-2	Prophylactic Antibiotic Selection for Surgical Patients
SCIP INF-3	Prophylactic Antibiotics Discontinued Within 24 Hours After Surgery End Time
SCIP INF-4	Cardiac Patients with Controlled 6 A.M. Postoperative Blood Glucose
SCIP INF-6	Surgery Patients with Appropriate Hair Removal
SCIP INF-9	Urinary Catheter Removed on Postoperative Day 1 (POD 1) or Postoperative Day 2 (POD 2) with Day of Surgery Being Day Zero
SCIP INF-10	Surgery Patients with Perioperative Temperature Management
SCIP CARD-2	Surgery Patients on Beta-Blocker Therapy Prior to Arrival Who Received a Beta-Blocker During the Perioperative Period
SCIP VTE-1	Surgery Patients with Recommended Venous Thromboembolism Prophylaxis Ordered
SCIP VTE-2	Surgery Patients Who Received Appropriate Venous Thromboembolism Prophylaxis Within 24 Hours Prior to Surgery to 24 Hours After Surgery

Fig. 1. Sample SCIP primer.

purpose (in this case, perioperative care).[6] A perioperative dashboard might include a process flowchart and unit performance data that are compared with national benchmarks and team goals for one or more SCIP measures.

Much like a primer, a dashboard must be developed, evaluated, and even reimagined by the key stakeholders and end users who make up the team. Dashboards can be powerful visual tools that can help teams highlight opportunities for process and/or performance improvement, celebrate surpassed benchmarks, and set new goals. **Fig. 2** is a sample dashboard of selected SCIP measures for a fictional hospital.

TWO LEARNING THEORIES
Knowles' Theory of Adult Learning

In his theory of adult learning, Knowles recognized that adult learners are pragmatic and self-directed (**Table 2**); they learn best when given opportunities to synthesize prior experience and new knowledge to solve real-life problems.[7] When bringing together the key stakeholders and end users to develop primers and dashboards for the perioperative setting, the real-life problem being addressed is the need for frontline nurses to understand, apply, and disseminate knowledge of SCIP measures. Perioperative nurses are not only responsible for meeting nurse-related responsibilities for SCIP protocols and benchmarks, they must also be knowledgeable enough to communicate them to nurses and clinicians from other teams who are also involved in the patient's continuity of care. In addition, as patient advocates, perioperative nurses also have a stake in ensuring that patient and caregiver preoperative and postoperative education on SCIP-related information is delivered accurately and effectively.

Vygotsky's Zone of Proximal Development

Although Vygotsky focused on child development, his theory of the zone of proximal development and the social process of learning has been applied across the

Dashboard for Selected SCIP Measures
January – April 2011

Surgical Case Mix (percent of total cases)

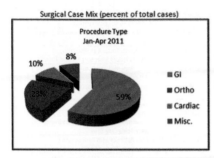

Average Antibiotic Prophylaxis Complete Times
Prior to Surgery (by patient type; 0-6 = 0-60 minutes)

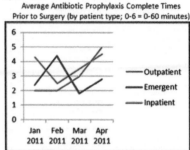

Number of Cases Exceeding 15-Minute Post-Op
Normothermia Standard (by procedure)

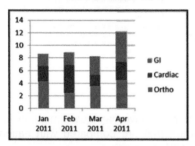

Number of Patients on β-Blocker at Admit
Who Received β-Blocker During Perioperative Period
(by procedure type; 0-5 = 0-50 patients)

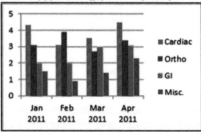

Fig. 2. Sample SCIP dashboard.

life span (see **Table 2**). Vygotsky believed that learning occurs only if two conditions are met:

1. Learning is triggered, developed, and refined only by interaction and cooperation with other people and the environment.
2. Learning occurs in the zone of proximal development, which is the gap between the learner's independent and potential problem-solving capability. To bridge that gap, the learner temporarily needs guidance and collaboration from peers who are more capable.[8]

Table 2 Comparing learning theories: Knowles and Vygotsky		
Theory	Knowles' Theory of Adult Learning	Vygotsky's Zone of Proximal Development
Population of interest	Adult learners	Children; however, theory has been applied to populations across life span
Population characteristics	Learners are pragmatic and self-directed	Learners are social
Phenomenon	Learning occurs when learners synthesize life experiences with new knowledge	Learning occurs in the zone of proximal development—gap between independent and potential problem-solving capability

In this way, learning is fundamentally a social activity. For perioperative nurse leaders tasked with the effort to track and benchmark unit, hospital, or system-level SCIP measures with dashboards, it is crucial to create an environment for frontline perioperative staff that allows adequate time for learning, applying, and mastering new knowledge, promotes social learning, and provides solid mentorship.

NEXT STEPS: TEACHING STRATEGIES

This section discusses suggested teaching strategies that use Knowles' and Vygotsky's principles of learning, with exemplars for consideration.

Create a Comfortable Psychological and Physical Environment that Facilitates Learning

According to Vygotsky, learning cannot occur without guidance and collaboration from experts committed to helping the learner navigate the knowledge gap.[8] *EXEMPLAR:* Introduce the idea of a perioperative nursing SCIP primer in a nonthreatening way to frontline nursing staff, such as advertising news of the initiative in a hospital or unit newsletter with an estimated target date for its availability to be reviewed by key stakeholders and end users.

Relate to Learners with Value and Respect for Their Feelings and Ideas

According to Knowles, adult learners believe they benefit most when they are allowed to draw from previous experiences during the learning process. This continued respect for the adult learner's life experience helps the learner feel valued.[7] *EXEMPLAR:* A proposed perioperative dashboard is introduced as a working draft, posted in a designated space and available for reviews and edits for an adequate amount of time. Several working meetings are scheduled for fielding suggestions and comments from key stakeholders and end users during the process of developing the dashboard so that as many people as possible have the opportunity to share their input.

Encourage Learners to Actively Participate in the Learning Activity

This strategy reflects Vygotsky's recognition that learning is a social activity—learners learn by listening, watching, learning from more experienced peers, sharing ideas with each other, and trying new things.[8] *EXEMPLAR:* Frontline perioperative staff and/or end users use the SCIP primer to help guide them in creating their first unit dashboard, with assistance from content experts available during scheduled meetings dedicated to team dashboard development. During these meetings, the goal is to establish a less formal (but still productive) working atmosphere that encourages learning while socializing.

Putting it All Together

Finally, it is important to help learners to make maximum use of their experiences within the learning process. This strategy reflects Vygotsky's learner in the zone of proximal development and Knowles' adult learner who synthesizes prior experience and new knowledge.[7,8] *EXEMPLAR:* Frontline perioperative nurses are able to connect data points and trends on their SCIP dashboards to specific care processes and outcomes. They participate regularly in reviewing, updating, and reimagining their team primer and dashboard, which now dovetails standards and data seamlessly.

REFERENCES

1. Centers for Medicare and Medicaid Services. National health expenditure data. Available at: https://www.cms.gov/nationalhealthexpenddata/02_nationalhealthaccountshistorical.asp. Accessed May 10, 2011.
2. Potenza B, Deligencia M, Estigoy B, et al. Lessons learned from the institution of Surgical Care Improvement Project at a teaching medical center. Am J Surg 2009;198:881–8.
3. Berenguer CM, Ochsner MG, Lord SA, et al. Improving surgical site infections: using National Surgical Quality Improvement Program Data to institute Surgical Care Improvement Project protocols in improving surgical outcomes. J Am Coll Surg 2010;210:737–41.
4. Edmiston CE, Spencer M, Lewis BD, et al. Reducing the risk of surgical site infections: did we really think SCIP was going to lead us to the promised land? Surg Infect (Larchmt) 2011;12:169–77.
5. Hawn MT, Vick CC, Richman J, et al. Surgical site infection prevention: time to move beyond the Surgical Care Improvement Program. Ann Surg 2011;254: 494–501.
6. Nelson EC, Batalden PB, Godfrey MM. Quality by design: a clinical microsystems approach. San Francisco: Wiley; 2007.
7. Knowles MS. The adult learner: a neglected species. 4th edition. Houston: Gulf; 1990.
8. Vygotsky LS. Mind in society: the development of higher psychological processes. Cambridge: Harvard; 1978.

Health Care Quality and Ethics
Implications for Practice and Leadership

Catherine Robichaux, PhD, RN, CCRN, CNS[a,*],
Jeanie Sauerland, BS, BSN, RN[b]

KEYWORDS

• Ethics principles • Virtue ethics • Care ethics • Patient care • Ethical climate

KEY POINTS

• This article proposes that ethics is the framework that supports quality and that nurses are central in this interdependence.
• Nurses have been involved with defining and assessing quality since long before the current emphasis on quality improvement and proliferation of quality/safety initiatives.
• The principles of autonomy, beneficence, nonmaleficence, and justice form the foundation of Western health care ethics, practice, and research.

INTRODUCTION

This article proposes that ethics is the framework that supports quality and that nurses are central in this interdependence. As Nelson and colleagues[1(p40)] maintain, "Quality care is built on ethical standards and ethical practices foster quality care." The requisites of quality care described by the Institute of Medicine (IOM) (patient-centered, safe, effective, timely, efficient, and equitable) embody ethical principles[1] and elements of both virtue and care ethics. To practice ethically and deliver quality care, nurses must work in a moral, caring environment that also reflects the same principles and qualities.

A brief history of the nursing profession's concern with quality and ethics is presented. A discussion of ethical principles, virtue ethics, and the ethics of care is provided, with examples of how they are manifested in the IOM quality aims. In addition, implications of the principles and virtue/care approaches for practice and leadership and their impact on quality care are suggested. An example is presented of ongoing collaboration between staff nurses and leadership to improve quality care through development of a nursing ethics council and unit-based ethics steward program.

[a] Department of Health Restoration and Systems Care Management, The University of Texas Health Science Center, 13156 Queens Forest, San Antonio, TX 78230, USA; [b] Nursing Ethics Committee, University Health System, 4502 Medical Drive, San Antonio, TX 78229, USA
* Corresponding author.
E-mail address: robichaux@uthscsa.edu

Perioperative Nursing Clinics 7 (2012) 333–342
http://dx.doi.org/10.1016/j.cpen.2012.06.002
1556-7931/12/$ – see front matter © 2012 Elsevier Inc. All rights reserved.

NURSING, QUALITY CARE, AND ETHICS: A BRIEF HISTORY

Nurses have been involved with defining and assessing quality since long before the current emphasis on quality improvement and proliferation of quality/safety initiatives. Florence Nightingale was responsible for perhaps the most remarkable hospital quality improvement ever undertaken and, as evident in her careful documentation, of both the processes and outcomes of care. Nightingale analyzed mortality data among British troops in 1855 at Scutari Hospital in what is now Istanbul and accomplished significant reductions in mortality through organizational and hygienic practices. She is also credited for creating in 1859 the world's first performance measures of hospitals. In 1974, Lang[2] proposed a quality assurance model that remains in use today. Based on societal and professional values as well as the most current scientific knowledge, Lang's work predates the IOM's definition of quality by almost 2 decades.

The quality mandate is also evident in standard 7 of *Nursing: The Scope and Standards of Practice*,[3] which states: "The registered nurse systematically enhances the quality and effectiveness of nursing practice." To accomplish this goal, the American Nurses' Association (ANA) has developed the National Database of Nursing Quality Indicators, which collects and evaluates unit-specific nurse-sensitive data from hospitals in the United States. The ANA has also established an online learning community for information on quality initiatives, the Nursing Quality Network.[4] In conjunction with the IOM, the Quality and Safety Education for Nurses[5] project endeavors to provide nurses with the knowledge, skills, and attitudes necessary to continuously improve the quality and safety of the health care systems in which they work.

Nurses also have an extensive history of identifying and responding to ethical issues in health care and taking seriously their moral responsibilities as health care practitioners. From the earliest nursing ethics text, *Hospital Sisters and their Duties* by Eva Luckes in 1886,[6] through the first ANA Code for Professional Nurses issued in 1926,[7] to development of the journal *Nursing Ethics* in 1994[8] and tenth revision of the *Code of Ethics for Nurses* in 2001,[9] nurses have continually sought to articulate their role as patient/family advocates and provide care based on ethical principles. Professional nursing organizations such as the Association of Perioperative Registered Nurses and the American Association of Critical Care Nurses (AACN) have published explications of the provisions of the code specifically for their respective members.[10,11] Both organizations, among others, have issued position statements and related documents on ethics and issues affecting quality care, including perioperative care of patients with do-not-resuscitate or allow-natural-death orders, patient safety, moral distress, and bullying/lateral violence.[12,13]

The essential, interdependent relationship between ethics and quality initiatives designed to measure, evaluate, and improve practice is contained in provision 3 of the *Codes of Ethics*, among others, and states: "The nurse promotes, advocates for, and strives to protect the health, safety, and rights of the patient."[9(p21)]

ETHICAL PRINCIPLES, VIRTUE AND CARE ETHICS, AND QUALITY

The principles of autonomy, beneficence, nonmaleficence, and justice form the foundation of Western health care ethics, practice, and research. These principles also "prescribe and justify nursing actions and form the basis for rules of behavior addressing patient-related issues such as informed consent, confidentiality, and veracity."[14] They also have implications for practice and leadership in regards to intraprofessional and interprofessional teamwork and developing an ethical climate in the perioperative area.

Unlike principle-based ethics, virtue ethics does not consist of fundamental rules for behavior but rather acknowledges the significance of moral character and the role of emotions and experiences in providing quality care. Virtue ethics involves a consistent, habitual pattern of perception, affective response, and action. Whereas ethical principles focus on "What should I do?" in a particular situation, virtue ethics asks "What kind of nurse should I be?"[15,16] As Dans[17] suggests, perhaps the greatest guarantee for quality health care for the patient lies in the character of the provider at both the practice and leadership levels. Virtues necessary for the provision of quality care in the perioperative area include prudence, compassion, veracity, and courage.

An ethic of care has particular relevance for health care quality because it recognizes the inherent relational nature of nursing practice. In this approach, patients and families are accepted and respected as unique individuals in situations that require interventions based on care, support, and sensitivity to context.[18] Milton[19(p110)] argues that inattention to situational context and a focus on "doing things right" rather than "doing the right thing" have the potential to harm the profession and those who receive our services. Milton suggests that the emphasis on quality and safety in the performance of nursing tasks and production of outcome evidence may diminish the meaning of the caring nurse-patient relationship. Milton questions whether the "monitoring for potential medical error is the new standard for nursing practice, rather than participating in the nurse-patient relationship with responsibility and accountability."

Supporting ethical principles with elements of virtue and care ethics may enable perioperative nurses to provide quality health care without losing the essential humanistic qualities that consistently make nursing the most trusted profession. This pluralist ethics approach may also contribute to development of an ethical environment in which nurses can practice quality care.

The relevance of ethical principles to the IOM quality aims and patient care are summarized in **Table 1**. They are discussed later in conjunction with virtue and care ethics. **Table 2** summarizes the implications of ethical principles, virtue, and care ethics for nursing practice and leadership, which are also discussed later.

AUTONOMY
Patient Care

In ethics, patient autonomy is the core of the concept of informed consent and dominates the relationship between patients and health care professionals. As noted in

Table 1 Ethics principles and quality of care		
Ethics Principles	**Application of Ethics Principles to Quality Aims**	**IOM's Quality Aims**
Autonomy	Supporting, facilitating and respecting self-determination in shared decision making	Patient-centered
Beneficence	Promoting the patient's beneficial health care and best interest	Effective, safe, timely, patient-centered
Nonmaleficence	Avoiding and protecting the patient from actions that cause harm	Safe, effective, patient-centered
Justice	Allocating fairly the benefits and burdens related to health care delivery and equitable access to health care services	Equitable, efficient, patient-centered

Reproduced from Nelson W, Gardent P, Shulman E, et al. Preventing ethics conflicts and improving healthcare quality through system redesign. Qual Saf Health Care 2010;19:527; with permission.

Table 2
Implications of ethics principles and virtue/care ethics to practice/leadership

Ethics Principles, Virtue, Care	Practice	Leadership
Autonomy	Autonomous decision-making, professional collaboration	Empowering governance structures
Beneficence	Treat one another with care/concern, assist our coworkers	Develop/sustain benevolent ethical climate
Nonmaleficence	Refrain from bullying/lateral violence	Adequate, competent staffing, provide communication/ assertiveness training
Justice	Treat coworkers with fairness/dignity	Develop a just culture; show interactional, informational, interpersonal justice
Virtue ethics	Compassion, veracity with coworkers	Veracity and dignity contribute to a just culture
Ethics of care	Collaborative relationships	Empathy and caring concern

Table 1, the IOM aim of patient-centered care promotes and respects patient autonomy. This aim focuses on shared decision making that includes provision of information that patients/families can comprehend and on presenting care/treatment options.[20,21] Respectful, compassionate communication elicits and considers patients' perspectives and promotes understanding of them as persons with guiding values. Although self-determination without undue influence may be key to patients' perceptions of quality care, it is enhanced by provider prudence. Understood as practical wisdom, prudence is considered a metavirtue because it is the one that must govern the other virtues. Prudence requires that perioperative nurses and all health care practitioners offer information regarding the availability, suitability, and cost of care.[22] Prudence also acknowledges that patients/families may need help in understanding what they believe and want in complex medical situations.[23]

Nurses understand that they must be sensitive to differences and shifts in patients' needs and wishes regarding their (patient's) autonomy. Promoting autonomy and ensuring quality care requires an in-depth knowledge of the patient in the context of the particular, caring situation.[24]

Implications for Practice and Leadership

In perioperative and all nursing practice, autonomy is defined as the freedom to make decisions within the domain of the profession and to act accordingly.[25] Professionalism is indicated by the ability to make autonomous decisions based on an extensive knowledge base, clinical expertise, and evidence.[26] Research indicates that inability to exercise autonomy in nursing practice is directly related to job dissatisfaction and perceptions of poor quality care. Limited nurse autonomy and poor intradisciplinary and interdisciplinary collaboration may also contribute to moral distress and intent to leave the job or profession.[27,28]

As summarized in **Table 2**, nurse autonomy is built on and enhanced through intraprofessional and interprofessional collaboration and active support by nursing leadership. Leaders show active support by being highly visible, providing praise and recognition, and including staff nurses on practice and operations committees. Supporting governance structures that empower perioperative nurses and promote cooperation shows respect for the concept of self-determination in nursing practice. Nurse managers can increase the safety and ethical climate of their units by facilitating an environment that enables nurses to provide care based on professional standards and in which they have a voice in quality/safety matters.[29,30]

NONMALEFICENCE

Nonmaleficence requires that health care professionals intentionally refrain from direct actions that would cause harm.[20] The current focus on preventing harm stems from the landmark IOM report *To Err is Human.*[31] This document indicated that more patients die each year from preventable medical errors than from traffic accidents, breast cancer, or the immunodeficiency virus. Although much has been accomplished in patient safety improvement since this report was issued, recent research suggests that patients remain at high risk for medical error.[32]

Reflecting the IOM quality aims of safe and patient-centered care (see **Table 1**), the principle of nonmaleficence also involves the obligation not to offer treatment that lacks efficacy. This obligation can become an issue in the provision of marginal, expensive, or scarce therapy in certain situations. Although the provision of treatment deemed nonefficacious is not an obligation for the health care professional, some patients and family members may believe it is their right to receive any treatment that they consider a potential benefit. This conflict frequently forms the basis for discussions of futility.[20]

Implications for Practice and Leadership

As patient and family advocates, perioperative nurses may experience moral distress when their voices are not heard and they are compelled to provide nonbeneficial or futile treatment. The virtues of moral courage, veracity, and compassion are essential in such situations. Lachman[33] defines moral courage as "the capacity to overcome fear and stand up for one's core values...the willingness to speak out in the face of forces that influence you to act in some other way." Moral courage is enhanced through development of ethical skills, including sensitivity and motivation, that enable the nurse to speak honestly and in a compassionate manner.[34] Moral courage and ethical skills serve to protect the patient from harm and preserve professional integrity.

Nurses must be able to provide safe care consistent with standards, adequate staffing, and competent team members. To maintain a quality, ethical environment, management and leadership must support nurse advocacy and role model speaking up and create cultures that support acts of courage in nursing.[35]

Although most nurses perceive their role as patient/family advocate as central in their practice, it may be less apparent in their treatment of one another. Research indicates that bullying and lateral violence are pervasive in all nursing areas and result in decreased quality of work, increased turnover, and diminished patient satisfaction. The reasons for such noncaring, harmful behaviors between or among nurses are varied; however, they seriously undermine the delivery of quality care.[36]

To overcome the harmful consequences of bullying and lateral violence, nurse leaders and managers should develop and enforce standards of behavior in their institutions. All staff must be made aware of which behaviors are acceptable at work and which are not and be held accountable for violations of the standards. Workshops focused on team training, communication, and assertiveness may also be offered to provide skills in preventing or overcoming negative workplace behaviors (see **Table 2**).[37]

BENEFICENCE

Beneficence and nonmaleficence are often discussed together, because the former is the performance of good acts that benefit others, whereas the latter requires avoiding actions that would harm oneself or others. Although both are important, the duty to do no harm is viewed as a stronger obligation in health care.[20] As noted in **Table 1**, their relationship to the IOM quality aims is similar. The distinction between the 2 lies in the fact that beneficence is a moral obligation to take positive steps to help others, not to simply prevent harm.[1] As discussed earlier, patients or family members may request a treatment or procedure that the professional believes will not be beneficial. In this case, they are not obligated to provide treatment that violates their conscience or professional integrity. On the other hand, patients and family members may refuse treatment that the provider deems beneficial.

Thompson[20] acknowledges that there is, at times, an inherent conflict between the principles of patient autonomy and beneficence. Although beneficence is an ancient concept found in the works of Aristotle, autonomy and the role of the patient in the decision-making process are paramount today. In this patient-centered model, paternalism, which implies coercion or deception through management of information by either not providing it or changing it, is not acceptable. The perioperative nurse's role in providing and clarifying information in a nonpaternalistic manner underscores the virtue of veracity in quality, patient-centered care.

Implications for Practice and Leadership

When applied to practice, beneficence means treating one another with care and concern and, as with patients, taking positive steps to help our peers (see **Table 2**). Recent research suggests that health care institutions and units that have benevolent, ethical climates may have better clinical outcomes, improved patient/family satisfaction, decreased mortality, and less nurse turnover.[38] The ethical climate is essentially a shared understanding of criteria that guide moral decision making in the workplace. Several types of ethical climate have been identified, including egoistic, principle, and benevolent, based on the primary criteria used for moral reasoning.[39]

In benevolent ethical climates, the nursing staff is supported in those decisions that benefit patients rather than the care team or themselves. Nurse leaders and managers can develop and sustain benevolent climates by encouraging staff to support one another and urging them to be concerned about how decisions and actions affect patients and the community. In a benevolent climate, teams are cohesive, discuss concerns, and develop interaction styles that support the group and patients. It might be assumed that ethical climates of health care organizations are benevolent. However, it is becoming more likely that nurses find their work environments to be punitive and defensive rather than focused on teamwork and delivery of quality care.[38,40]

JUSTICE

Thompson[20] observes that many terms have been used to describe the ethical principle of justice, including fairness and entitlement. He also notes that there are several types and theories of justice, including that of distributive justice, which is included in **Table 1**. The ethical principle of distributive justice underlies current debates on the affordable care act, insurance mandates, health care access, and equitable care. In **Table 1**, justice encompasses the IOM quality aims of equitable, efficient, and, as with all aims, patient-centered.

Nurses are required by the ANA Code of Ethics to provide fair and equal treatment that respects the "inherent dignity, worth, and uniqueness of every individual, unrestricted by considerations of social or economic status, personal attributes, or the nature of the health problem."[9(p7)] Further, the just provision of care requires these factors be considered, because they influence the need for care and the allocation of health care resources. This idea expands what is addressed in the IOM quality aim (see **Table 1**), because the notion of social justice is also recognized.

Daily patient care issues affected by the principle of distributive justice include those of rationing, allocation, and use of scarce resources. Nurses may ration care activities because of insufficient time or inadequate staffing.[41] Identified care activities rationed include discharge planning, teaching and comforting. The effects of such rationing on quality care and patient outcomes have not been sufficiently studied. However, preliminary results indicate that those nurses who had to ration care reported higher levels of job dissatisfaction and emotional exhaustion. The virtue of prudence has application for the often necessary rationing of perioperative nursing care activities. This practical wisdom, gained through experience, enables nurses to safely balance complex and competing care demands.

Implications for Practice and Leadership

As with patients, nurses are required to treat coworkers with justice and dignity regardless of personal attributes (see **Table 2**). There is a long history of resentment between nurses with different educational preparation and reports of bullying/lateral violence between nurses from different cultures. Aside from being personally harmful, these behaviors are considered unfair and can affect the quality of patient care. Fairness and justice are closely intertwined and 1 term is often used to describe the other. Impartiality, veracity, and nonbias are behaviors associated with justice.

Nurse leaders and managers are responsible for creating a just culture in the perioperative area and elsewhere. Morrow[37(p191)] describes a just culture as one in which "patient safety is promoted through encouraging employees to disclose incidences that are out of the ordinary and/or errors that they have missed or discovered." Morrow maintains that this behavior does not encourage a "blameless culture" but rather one that balances human error with human safety and treats all involved with fairness. Squires and colleagues[42] reported that nurse leaders who showed interactional justice, synonymous with fairness, combined with informational justice (the provision of adequate, timely, honest, and complete information) and interpersonal justice (being treated with respect and dignity during interactions) contributed to increased safety climate outcomes (see **Table 2**). Safety climate is defined as the current state of employees' actions and behaviors that reflects the fundamental safety culture. It shows the employees' perceptions of safety policies, procedures and practices in use within an organization and acts as a frame of reference for their behavior and attitudes.[43]

AN EXAMPLE OF PRACTICE/LEADERSHIP COLLABORATION TO IMPROVE HEALTH CARE QUALITY

University Health System (UHS) in San Antonio, Texas, is a safety-net facility serving a predominantly underserved population. Before Magnet designation and subsequent recommendations, the perioperative nurse educator (JS) was concerned about the many ethically challenging situations in that area and others. She questioned her role in the decision-making process and wondered whether other nurses shared her concerns about doing the ethically right thing for patients and families. Many of the nurses she spoke to appeared to lack knowledge about what constituted an ethical situation. When an ethical situation was recognized, many nurses did not know how to proceed or how to obtain an ethics consult. Consequently, JS developed a presentation on basic ethics concepts and the steps involved in obtaining an ethics consult at UHS. She shared her presentation with other nurse educators and at the Magnet workshops.

An appraisal visit by Magnet consultants raised several concerns regarding nurses' role in ethical issues and ethical decision making, including which ethical issues were of concern at UHS, who addressed ethical issues at UHS, who was allowed to serve on the bioethics committee and what was their role, and what education bioethics committee members received.

Although JS had anecdotal reports about the ethical concerns at UHS, she and the Magnet Director determined that they would require research-based findings to move the ethics project forward. They and several other interested staff nurses and nurse educators enlisted the skills of a faculty mentor (CR) to conduct a mixed-methods study exploring registered nurse moral distress and ethical climate at UHS. Nurses (N = 360) from throughout the facility, including the perioperative area, participated in completing 2 online surveys and responded to 2 open-ended questions. Survey results indicated that nurses were experiencing moderate levels of moral distress, especially in regard to perceived incompetence of various health care providers (nurse assistants, registered nurses, physicians) and inadequate staffing. Higher levels of moral distress were associated with diminished perceptions of ethical climate, which was rated moderately, overall. Responses to the open-ended questions provided additional insights into causes of moral distress and diminished ethical climate, including situations of bullying and lateral violence, The findings from the moral distress/ethical climate study were shared with the Chief Nursing Officer, who agreed to provide support for development of a nursing ethics council and unit-based ethics steward program.

The nursing ethics council is unique in that it has relevance for all shared governance councils at UHS. Members represent most units in UHS, including the perioperative area, and serve a 3-year term. The council meets monthly and has members from other disciplines, such as child life. Agenda items are based on concerns or ethics educational needs of the members who meet monthly. Various members, invited guests, a nursing faculty mentor, the bioethics committee chairperson, and a nurse lawyer provide ongoing ethics education at monthly meetings. Social workers, pastoral care, physical therapists, and physicians have also attended the meetings. An annual all-day ethics conference provides additional educational opportunities for the health care community regarding ethical issues such as bullying and conflict resolution. Nursing ethics council members serve as ethics stewards for their respective units and are a resource regarding ethics concerns and questions. The cochairs of the nursing ethics council also serve on the institutional bioethics committee.

The nursing ethics council and ethics steward program have been in existence for approximately 3 years and their effects on improving health care quality are continuing. There has been a substantial increase in ethics consults, establishment of pain management protocols, and increased awareness of the detrimental effects of bullying. Members of the council have presented their research findings at the ANA Nursing Ethics Conference and will share development of the council and ethics stewards program at the upcoming AACN educational meeting in 2012.

This practice/leadership collaboration represents efforts to establish a just culture and a caring, benevolent ethical climate. Developing a collaborative practice environment that values veracity and the relevance of ethics principles, virtue, and care ethics in patient care and in professional relationships serves to enhance health care quality.

REFERENCES

1. Nelson W, Gardent P, Shulman E, et al. Preventing ethics conflicts and improving healthcare quality through system redesign. Qual Saf Health Care 2010;19: 526–30.
2. Mitchell P. Defining patient safety and quality care (Prepared with support from the Robert Wood Johnson Foundation). AHRQ Publication No. 08-0043. In: Hughes R, editor. Patient safety and quality: an evidence-based handbook for nurses. Rockville (MD): Agency for Healthcare Research and Quality; 2008. p. 1–5.
3. American Nurses' Association. Nursing: scope and standards of practice. 2nd edition. Silver Springs (MD): American Nurses' Association; 2010.
4. Montalvo I. The national database of nursing quality indicators (NDNQI). Online J Issues Nurs 2007;12:3.
5. Cronenwett L, Sherwood G, Barnsteiner J, et al. Quality and safety education for nurses. Nurs Outlook 2007;55:122–31.
6. Luckes E. Hospital sisters and their duties. Philadelphia: P. Blakiston Son & Co; 1886.
7. American Nurses' Association. A suggested code: a code of ethics presented for the consideration of the American Nurses' Association. Am J Nurs 1926;26: 599–600.
8. Tschudin V, Hunt G. Nursing development units. Nurs Ethics 1994;1:1–2.
9. American Nurses' Association. Code of ethics for nurses with interpretive statements. Silver Springs (MD): American Nurses' Association; 2001.
10. Seifert P. The ANA code of ethics and AORN's explications. Periop Nurse Clinics 2008;3:183–9.
11. Kline A. ANA code of ethics for nurses: provision stresses advocate role. AACN News. May 2005: 22.
12. Association of Perioperative Nurses. Position statements on patient safety and healthy perioperative work environment. 2011. Available at: http://www.aorn.org/PracticeResources/AORNPositionStatements/. Accessed February 12, 2012.
13. American Association of Critical Care Nurses. Position statement on moral distress. 2008. Available at: http://www.aacn.org/WD/Practice/Docs/Moral_Distress.pdf. Accessed February 12, 2012.
14. Volbrecht R. Nursing ethics: communities in dialogue. Upper Saddle River (NJ): Prentice-Hall; 2002.
15. Armstrong A. Toward a strong virtue ethics for nursing practice. Nurs Philos 2006; 7:110–24.
16. Austin W. The terminal: a tale of virtue. Nurs Philos 2007;7:54–61.
17. Dans PE. Clinical peer review: burnishing a tarnished icon. Ann Intern Med 1993; 118:566–8.
18. Watson J. Nursing: human science and human care. Sudbury (MA): Jones & Bartlett; 1999.
19. Milton C. An ethical exploration of quality and safety initiatives in nursing practice. Nurs Sci Q 2011;24:107–10.
20. Thompson D. Principles of ethics: in managing a critical care unit. Crit Care Med 2007;35:S2–10.
21. Nelson A. Ethics: a foundation for quality. Healthc Exec 2011;22:46–9.
22. Huycke L, Hall A. Quality in healthcare and ethical principles. J Adv Nurs 2000; 32:562–71.
23. Epstein R, Peters E. Beyond information: exploring patients' preferences. JAMA 2009;302(2):195–7.

24. Moser A, Houtepen R, Widdershoven G. Patient autonomy in nurse-led shared care: a review of theoretical and empirical literature. J Adv Nurs 2007;57(4):357–65.

25. Weston MJ. Strategies for enhancing autonomy and control over nursing practice. Online J Issues Nurs 2010. Available at: http:www.nursingworld.org/MainMenuCategories/ANAMarketplace/ANAPeriodicals/OJIN/TableofContents/Vol15210/No1Jan2010/Enhancing-Autonomy-and-Control-and-Practice.html.

26. Papathanassoglou E, Katanikola E, Kalafati M, et al. Professional autonomy, collaboration with physicians, and moral distress among European intensive care nurses. Am J Crit Care 2012;21:41–52.

27. Baggs JG, Schmitt MH, Mushlin AI, et al. Association between nurse-physician collaboration and patient outcomes in three intensive care units. Crit Care Med 1999;27(9):1992–8.

28. Manojlovich M, Antonakos CL, Ronis DL. Intensive care units, communication between nurses and physicians, and patients' outcomes. Am J Crit Care 2009; 18(1):21–30.

29. Hofmeyer A, Marck P. Building social capital in healthcare organizations: thinking ecologically for safer care. Nurs Outlook 2008;56:145–51.

30. Stone P, Hughes R, Dailey M. Creating a safe and high quality healthcare environment (Prepared with support from the Robert Wood Johnson Foundation). AHRQ Publication No. 08-0043. In: Hughes R, editor. Patient safety and quality: an evidence-based handbook for nurses. Rockville (MD): Agency for Healthcare Research and Quality; 2008. p. 1–5.

31. Institute of Medicine. To err is human: building a safer health system. 2000. Available at: http://www.nap.edu/catalog.php?record_id=9728. Accessed February 12, 2012.

32. Agency for Healthcare Policy and Research. Patient safety: one decade after to err is human. 2009. Available at: http://www.psqh.com/septemberoctober-2009/234-september-october-2009-ahrq.html. Accessed February 12, 2012.

33. Lachman V. Patient safety: the ethical imperative. Medsurg Nurs 2007;16:401–3.

34. Robichaux C. Developing ethical skills: from sensitivity to action. Crit Care Nurse 2012;32:65–72.

35. LaSala C, Bjarnason D. Creating workplace environments that support moral courage. Online J Issues Nurs 2010. Available at: http://www.nursingworld.org/MainMenuCategories/EthicalStandards/Courage-and-Distress/Workplace-Environments. Accessed March 3, 2012.

36. Lindy C, Schaefer F. Negative workplace behaviors: an ethical dilemma for nurse managers. J Nurs Manag 2010;18:295–302.

37. Morrow M. Fairness and justice in leading-following: opportunities to foster integrity in first 100 days. Nurs Sci Q 2012;25:188–93.

38. Rathert C, Fleming D. Hospital ethical climate and teamwork in acute care: the moderating role of leaders. Health Care Manage Rev 2008;33(4):323–31.

39. Victor B, Cullen J. The organizational bases of ethical work climates. Adm Sci Q 1988;33:101–25.

40. Robichaux C, Parsons M. An ethical framework for developing and sustaining a healthy workplace. Crit Care Nurs Q 2009;32(3):199–207.

41. Rochefort C, Clarke S. Nurses' work environments, care rationing, job outcomes, and quality of care on neonatal units. J Adv Nurs 2010;66(10):2213–24.

42. Squires M, Tourangeau A, Spence H, et al. The link between leadership and safety outcomes in hospitals. J Nurs Manag 2010;18:914–25.

43. Clarke S. The relationship between safety climate and safety performance: a meta-analytic review. J Occup Health Psychol 2006;11(4):315–27.

The Role of the Clinical Nurse Specialist in the Future of Health Care in the United States

Jacqueline M. Gordon, MSN, RN, CCNS, CCRN[a],
Jennifer D. Lorilla, MSN, RN, United States Army Nurse Corps[b],
Cheryl A. Lehman, PhD, RN, CNS-BC, RN-BC, CRRN[c],*

KEYWORDS

- Clinical nurse specialist • CNS • APRN • Licensed independent practitioner
- Licensed independent provider

KEY POINTS

- The needs of the health care system and expectations of health care consumers can be met by an exceptionally trained Advanced Practice Registered Nurse (APRN): the clinical nurse specialist (CNS).
- However, role confusion related to the CNS, by developing competing roles that do not have APRN privileges, has created challenges for current and future CNSs to overcome.
- CNSs in the United States have consistently documented outcomes including improved quality of care, decreased costs, and improved patient satisfaction.

INTRODUCTION

The Clinical Nurse Specialist (CNS) has the potential to play a large and important role in assuring the delivery of high-quality health services to the citizens of the United States, but has often struggled with attaining recognition, reimbursement, and regard as an Advanced Practice Registered Nurse (APRN). The health care industry does not always seem to understand the value and potential of the CNS, in part attributable to the varied roles the CNS may play, such as independent licensed provider, clinical

---

The views expressed in this abstract/manuscript are those of the author(s) and do not reflect the official policy or position of the Department of the Army, Department of Defense, or the US Government.
[a] Heart and Vascular Institute, Penn State Hershey Medical Center, Hershey, PA 17033, USA;
[b] Department of Medicine, Tripler Army Medical Center, 1 Jarrett White Road, Tripler AMC, Hawaii 96859, USA; [c] Department of Health Restoration and Care Systems Management, School of Nursing, The University of Texas Health Science Center at San Antonio, MC 7975, 7703 Floyd Curl Drive, San Antonio, TX 78229-3900, USA
* Corresponding author.
E-mail address: lehmanc@uthscsa.edu

Perioperative Nursing Clinics 7 (2012) 343–353
http://dx.doi.org/10.1016/j.cpen.2012.06.006
1556-7931/12/$ – see front matter © 2012 Elsevier Inc. All rights reserved.

expert and nurse educator. Some markets limit the CNS to a single role (typically, the nurse educator), whereas others use the CNS to their fullest potential as clinical expert, involving their CNS employees in quality monitoring and improvement, implementation of evidence-based practices in the workplace, and as expert clinical practitioners in varied settings including primary, secondary, and tertiary care. This article explores the future of the CNS in health care in the United States.

HISTORICAL PERSPECTIVE

The CNS is 1 of 4 recognized APRN roles in the United States: the CNS, the Nurse Practitioner (NP), the Certified Nurse Midwife (CNM), and the Certified Nurse Anesthetist (CRNA). Under state-specific rules and regulations, the CNS has the ability and training to medically diagnose and manage the patient as an independent licensed provider; to prescribe medications, including scheduled drugs; to work as an expert nurse within systems to monitor and improve the quality of care; to provide training to practicing nurses and other providers; to collaborate with and/or lead the interprofessional team in team efforts such as program development; and to attend to the myriad of clinical patient, nurse, and systems issues that permeate the everyday world of the health care institution.

The use of the term "specialist" in nursing emerged in the 1900s. An article published in the first issue of the *American Journal of Nursing* entitled "Specialties in Nursing" noted the importance of specialty practice amongst nurses.[1] Psychiatric nursing was the first nursing specialty; originating from the Quaker reformers who challenged the brutal treatment of the insane and advocated for gentler methods of social control in the second half of the nineteenth century.[2] The CNS role grew substantially in the following decades. The American Nurses Association (ANA) officially recognized the CNS as an expert practitioner in 1974 and included master's education as a requirement for the CNS.[2] The first state to recognize diagnosis and treatment as part of the scope of practice of specialty nurses was Idaho in 1971.[2] At this time boards of medicine and nursing met and developed regulations for practice.[3]

In the 1980s, requirements were instituted for nurses wishing to assume the title of CNS. The ANA's Social Policy Statement stated that to use the title CNS, study and supervised clinical practice must occur at the graduate level of education and requirements should be met for specialty certification through nursing's professional society.[4] In the early 1980s, CNSs were sought after and new training programs were being demanded. By 1984 the National League for Nursing had accredited 129 programs for preparation of the CNS.[2] By the end of the 1980s and beginning of the 1990s cost containment became a priority of the health care industry, and CNSs shifted away from being bedside expert clinicians toward administrator roles or staff educators, as a result of budget cutbacks.[2] However, in 1995 the National Association of Clinical Nurse Specialists (NACNS) was established, and CNSs were subsequently identified for Medicare reimbursement eligibility in 1997.[2] Organizational development of CNSs and legal inclusion of the CNS in reimbursement during the 1990s were vital to the continuation of the CNS role.

The CNS has regained support in recent years because of the noted contribution of the CNS to health care systems. The Institute of Medicine (IOM) has released reports focusing on the need for increased quality and safety in health care.[5] The CNS plays a pivotal role in quality improvement, patient safety, and improved health care outcomes, and continues to deserve a place in the future of health care in the United States.

DEFINING THE CNS

The NACNS has released numerous publications regarding the CNS role.[6,7] The NACNS's Statement on Clinical Nurse Specialist Practice and Education[7] clearly defines the role of the CNS. Historically the CNS role has been further divided into subroles such as direct patient care provider, consultant, educator, researcher, collaborator, and clinical leader[8]; however, it was determined that this framework for CNS practice did little to distinguish the CNS from other nursing roles.[9] NACNS defines CNSs as:

> Licensed registered professional nurses with graduate preparation...from a program that prepares CNSs. They may also be prepared in a post-master's certificate program that is recognized by a national nursing accrediting body as preparing graduates to practice as a CNS for a specialty population...CNSs are clinical experts in the diagnosis and treatment of illness, and the delivery of evidence-based nursing interventions...CNSs work with other nurses to advance their nursing practices and improve outcomes, and provide clinical expertise to effect system-wide changes to improve programs of care.[7]

CNS areas of specialization can be based on population (eg, pediatric), type of problem (eg, surgical), setting (eg, inpatient), type of care (eg, critical care), or disease/pathology/medical specialty (eg, spinal cord injury, cardiac, pulmonary).[7] CNS practice competencies are applied to 3 interacting spheres of influence: the patient/client sphere, the nurses/nursing sphere, and the organization/system sphere.[7] CNS practice then occurs within the specialty chosen by that particular CNS in which core competencies are enacted.

CNS COMPETENCIES

CNSs enact the following 8 core competencies regardless of specialty or setting.[7]

1. Using "knowledge of differential illness diagnoses and treatments in comprehensive, holistic assessments of patients within the context of disease, diagnoses, and treatments."
2. Providing innovative interventions to achieve quality, cost-effective nurse-sensitive outcomes by designing, implementing, and evaluating individual and/or population-based programs.
3. Serving "as a leader/consultant/mentor/change agent in advancing the practice of nursing among other nurses and across organizations to achieve outcomes."
4. Advancing nursing practice by applying evidence-based interventions, using best-practice guidelines, and modifying professional standards and policies that direct care of nursing personnel and other providers of health care to improve outcomes.
5. Acting as a leader for interprofessional groups to facilitate collaboration with other disciplines in the attainment of outcomes across the continuum of care.
6. Identifying resource needs at the system level for delivery of nursing care, and attaining those resources.
7. Helping to "expand the practice of nursing through ongoing generation and acquisition of scientific knowledge and skills to maintain expert clinical competencies that leads to desired outcomes."
8. Demonstrating "professional citizenship and fiscal responsibility in the health care system by focusing on health policy and/or resource management to ensure quality, cost-effective outcomes of nursing care."

CNS EDUCATION

CNS training, as already mentioned, is at the master's level. It includes courses in advanced pathophysiology, advanced pharmacology, and advanced health assessment, as well as courses in medical diagnosis and management, CNS role, nursing theory, research, and evidence-based practice.

In addition to the core requirements, NACNS recommends that the following additional core content specific to CNS practice be included in CNS educational programs:

- Theoretical foundations for CNS practice
- Theoretical and empiric knowledge of phenomena of concern that forms the basis for assessment, diagnosis, and treatment of illness and wellness
- Theoretical and scientific base for the design and development of innovative nursing interventions
- Clinical inquiry/critical thinking with advanced knowledge
- Selection, use, and evaluation of technology/products/devices
- Theories of teaching, mentoring, and coaching in all 3 spheres
- Influencing change
- Systems thinking
- Leadership development for interprofessional collaboration
- Consultation theory
- Measurement
- Evidence-based practice and research use[7]

CNS programs of study also include clinical experiences, with a preceptorship that includes at least 500 clinical hours. Ensuring that CNSs are educated based on the curriculum outlined by the NACNS is essential to producing well-prepared CNSs upon entry into practice.

CURRENT STATE: THE CNS AND SOCIETAL NEEDS

CNSs have the ability and training to function in several roles, including those as provider of patient care at an advanced level (ie, independent licensed provider) and as an advanced practice nurse within a health care system, educating staff, ensuring quality, and monitoring care. Patients, nurses, and health care institutions all have needs that the CNS can address. These needs include, among others: improving access to care for all populations; ensuring the delivery of high-quality, safe health care; meeting requirements of accrediting agencies; evaluating the best evidence and putting it into practice; educating nursing students and nurses; procuring safe, effective, and efficient equipment for patient care; and developing health care programs to meet population needs.

Independently Licensed Provider Role

With the Affordable Care Act (ACA) being signed into law in March 2010, the opportunity for transforming health care in the United States is both imminent and ongoing. The prospect of providing health care that is of higher quality, safer, more affordable, and more accessible is appealing. However, it is suspected that with the passage of the ACA an additional 32 million previously uninsured Americans will be seeking health care services.[10] Who will care for these newly insured patients? Access to care has been an established long-term issue in the United States and has increased since the advent of the ACA. Physicians cannot carry the sole burden of caring for the increasing number of patients. APRNs such as CNSs can help bridge the gap and aid people in accessing health care in the United States if CNSs are allowed to practice to their fullest ability.

In the 1990s, federal regulations were enacted allowing Medicare reimbursement for CNSs that had been previously omitted.[2] CNSs are now practicing around the nation in a multitude of environments such as primary care clinics, intensive care units, and specialty clinics, and are able to bill for their services. At present, scope of practice including prescriptive authority is regulated by each specific state Board of Nursing (BON). Each state is able to mandate restrictions on CNS practice. Some of these limitations include geographic distance between supervising physician and CNS, number of charts a supervising physician must review on a monthly basis, and number of advanced practice nurses (eg, CNSs and NPs) per supervising physician.[10]

For those CNSs practicing as independently licensed providers who bill Medicare, Medicare's definition of a CNS for billing purposes states that a CNS is:

- A registered nurse (RN) currently licensed to practice in the State where he or she practices and is authorized to furnish the services of a CNS in accordance with state law
- Has a Master of Science in Nursing or Doctor of Nursing Practice (DNP) in a defined clinical area of nursing from an accredited educational institution
- Is certified as a CNS by a recognized national certifying body that has established standards for CNSs

Medicare will pay CNSs if they meet Medicare qualification requirements and the practice or facility accepts Medicare payments, which is reimbursed at 85% of the Medicare Physician fee schedule amount. Medicare also has inpatient hospital billing principles, which in part state that the billed services must be a physician service, medically necessary, within the CNS scope of practice, and documented as required. Thus, qualified CNSs can be helpful to the hospital's bottom line by billing for services delivered in the inpatient as well as the outpatient setting.[11]

Legislative restrictions related to APRN practice often create decreased access to care. In reality, in salary and benefits CNSs and all APRNs cost less than physicians. Preparing an APRN in comparison with a physician requires less time and less expense, and education is less lengthy and less expensive than that of physicians. The IOM recommended in 2011 in the report *The Future of Nursing: Leading Change, Advancing Health* that APRNs should be able to practice to the full extent of their education and training.[12] The IOM recommended actions for Congress to take, consisting of expanding the Medicare program to include coverage of APRN services that are within the scope of practice under applicable state law, just as physician services are now covered. The report further recommends that state legislatures reform scope of practice regulations to conform to the National Council of State Boards of Nursing APRN model rules and regulations. By allowing APRNs to practice to the full extent of their education and training, access to health care and primary care barriers can be surmounted.

CNSs have been proved to provide care at a lower cost than care provided by physicians, and a high level of evidence supports use of the CNS role to decrease the costs of care.[13] One recent randomized controlled trial identified that cost savings were achieved by substituting physicians with diabetes nurse specialists in caring for patients with diabetes.[14] The CNS has a very important role to play in providing care as an independent licensed provider, especially with regard to underserved populations, and should certainly be used within this role to improve access to health care in the United States.

Institutionally Focused Roles

In addition to providing a bridge to the gap of access to care, the CNS is essential within our health care institutions. Potential roles for the CNS within an institution include expert clinician, nurse educator, interprofessional team leader, consultant, quality monitor, and champion of evidence-based practice.

For example, facilities receiving Magnet designation through the American Nurses Credentialing Center (ANCC) are highly revered, and have been proven to provide high-quality nursing care and exceptional processes for the delivery of nursing care. Clinical practice change and sustained process improvement are foundations of Magnet designation, and CNSs have the ideal skill set to make these impacts occur at a systems level and to aid in obtaining and sustaining Magnet recognition.[15]

CNSs often serve as nurse educator within institutions, ensuring that staff is current in knowledge. As a nurse educator, the CNS does more than provide required education for staff. The CNS conducts needs assessments of staff, examining national trends in care of the patient population, the latest evidence in medical and nursing care, the latest equipment purchases, the recent quality issues, patient comments, and other quality data to plan educational interventions that meet the needs of both the staff and the patients. The CNS then conducts outcome studies related to the education provided: did it make a difference and how?

CNSs also participate in education to train new nurses. A recent editorial by Gerard[16] reflects on her experience as a student in a baccalaureate nursing program. Students were educated by master's and doctorally prepared CNSs using the unification model of education that combined teaching with clinical practice, research, and/or administration. Gerard learned to respect the CNS practitioner-teachers and saw that nurses, medical interns, and residents recognized them as the "go-to" experts driven by their expert knowledge and high quality of practice. CNSs taught students to be a role model and to participate in multidisciplinary meetings to improve plans of care for patients and to participate in professional organizations and meetings with government officials; guided students through systems-level thinking to support a safe environment and promote a high quality of care; and involved them in acquiring knowledge, research, and evaluating evidence. While education by CNS faculty are certainly measurable as outcomes such as graduation rates and NCLEX (National Council Licensure Examination) scores, CNSs who teach in schools of nursing also make immeasurable differences in the students they teach.

In recent years, specialty programs such as heart failure clinics and palliative care teams have become more popular. CNSs are emerging as leaders in the specialty fields that include programs certified by The Joint Commission (TJC), such as stroke centers. The TJC has also added advanced institutional certifications for other specialties including diabetes, ventricular assist devices, chronic kidney disease, and hip fracture. The CNS is the ideal APRN to aid facilities in obtaining this type of recognition while providing clinical expertise in the specialty areas.

CNS OUTCOMES

Outcomes such as improved quality of care can be directly related to CNS practice. The Centers for Medicare and Medicaid Services (CMS) has proposed a new system of reimbursement for hospitals that uses a value-based purchasing strategy based on quality data for annual repayment.[17] The CNS within an institution can be instrumental in instituting tracking measures and procedural changes to improve quality of care and obtain maximal reimbursement.[18] CNSs can implement strategies using evidence-based practice to improve quality of care and decrease costs. Optimal outcomes are synonymous with CNS practice.

The literature abounds with examples of the differences that the CNS can make in today's health care environment. Reductions in cost, length of stay, patient complications, and rehospitalizations, increases in patient satisfaction and quality of life, successful formation of new programs, and attainment of quality goals have all been attributed to CNS practice. The difference is apparent not only in patient outcomes, but also manifests in staff-centered interventions such as back safety programs that reduce cost and staff injury[19] and the facilitation of evidence-based practice.[18]

The literature review by Moore and McQuestion[20] presents an excellent summary of the role of the CNS in chronic disease management. A sample of CNS outcomes in this review include decreased rehospitalizations, shorter lengths of stay, lower hospital costs, improved quality of life for patients, and improvements in patient function, all of which are valuable to health care institutions in today's financial picture. Mahler[21] describes the CNS role in development of a geropalliative model of care at a large health care facility. The CNS's role on the team was to influence the practice of nursing staff, and to be a nursing mentor, consultant, and educator.

Another example of CNS outcomes is the Cancer Reform Strategy, which recognized the importance of the CNS in improving the experience of patients diagnosed with cancer.[22] The findings of this study demonstrated that CNS involvement improved patients' experience and satisfaction with the breast cancer service. As a result of the CNS role in the breast cancer service, the CNS had a visible role to patients as a consultant and was enabled to meet the informational needs of patients, assess their nursing needs, and support them through their treatment. The CNS's ability to coordinate care and provide appropriate and timely information, social and psychological support, and continuity of care enhanced the patients' experience through such a difficult time.

The Hospital of the University of Pennsylvania has operationalized unit-based CNS-related outcomes into a CNS scorecard. This scorecard tracks outcomes at the unit level that can be influenced by the CNS, such as urinary tract infections, ventilator-associated pneumonia, bloodstream infections, pressure ulcers, and falls, as well as staff knowledge levels, patient satisfaction, promotion of evidence-based practices, and staff turnover and satisfaction.[23] The advantage of such a scorecard is that it allows the CNS to focus on issues important to the setting and the patients, and also communicates to others the importance of the CNS in affecting these outcomes.

APPLICATION OF CNS PRACTICE

Operationalizing the CNS role can be challenging. Two CNSs in the authors' own community are actively engaged in the CNS role at a local teaching hospital's intensive care unit (ICU). These CNSs have received accolades from the nurses they work with, physicians, and supervisors for their excellence in care and their importance to the organization. Recently they shared some examples of successful implementation of CNS practice.

The first CNS was able to change the culture in the medical ICU. Both physicians and nursing staff commented that before the CNS arrived, communication was poor and cohesiveness was absent. With his presence on daily interprofessional rounds, this CNS encouraged nurses on his unit to voice their concerns related to patient care, thus opening the door for better communication, improved teamwork, mutual respect, and collaboration among staff. He states that CNS presence empowered the nurses to believe that they could openly communicate with the team because they felt that the CNS was their advocate. Physicians are also appreciative that the CNS serves as consultant, expert clinician, and educator by providing on-the-spot training, while avoiding near misses, and improving patient outcomes through application of clinical knowledge and expertise.

Another example from this CNS concerns the introduction of an electromagnetic device used to safely insert feeding tubes at the bedside. Before implementation of the device, physicians were the only staff members allowed to place enteral feeding tubes for patients. After research and buy-in from the medical director and nurses, the CNS was able to develop and implement a clinical practice guideline that allowed nursing to place enteral feeding tubes after training, and 5 successful Dobhoff enteral feeding tube placements using the electromagnetic placement device. With the addition of a new and necessary nursing skill, the physicians were freed from placing feeding tubes and the nurses were able to add to their scope of practice.

The second CNS is currently involved in implementation of a mobility protocol, an evidence-based protocol to get ICU patients who meet criteria out of bed and walking while on a ventilator. This protocol encourages early mobility of ventilated patients and improves patient outcomes by increasing patients' well-being, function, and number of days out of bed while decreasing time spent on a ventilator and length of stay in the ICU and hospital, as well as decreasing delirium and dosages of narcotics and benzodiazepines. The mobility protocol was introduced by a physician, and the CNS served as a representative for nursing. She researched the nursing literature on mobility, and ensured that nursing concerns were addressed and incorporated into the protocol. She included bedside nurses in protocol development to ensure that the protocol was feasible and safe, and to get the initial buy-in. It has been almost 7 months since the initial trial. One of the nurses on the team recently attended the National Teaching Institute, a nursing educational conference, and attended all the lectures and posters that addressed mobility to evaluate their strategies and lessons learned; which has led to a mobility reinvigoration campaign. The CNS's goal is for nursing to own this protocol and spread this to other units for implementation.

This CNS is also involved in nursing research at the facility. She was consulted by a bedside nurse to assist with development of a study comparing penlight and pupillometer methods of pupil assessment. The CNS and the nurse searched together for articles on the subject matter and proceeded from there. The CNS also authored the Institutional Review Board protocol in keeping with the vision of the study. This study is still ongoing and is evaluating its outcomes.

Many CNSs in the authors' community are engaged in the role of independent licensed provider. Some of the sites are private clinics in a physician practice, such as vascular and cardiology, where they follow their own assigned patients. Others work on physician teams in ICUs, trauma clinics, and emergency rooms, where they see patients and also supervise the work of the medical residents. Some CNSs follow patients both in the clinic and in the hospital, assessing, diagnosing, and prescribing medications across the continuum of care. Some lead programs, such as heart failure clinics and stroke centers of excellence. Many of these CNSs serve as preceptors for CNS students, NP students, and even medical students.

All of these CNSs are recognized as key players in their facilities, and many are leaders at the national level. These CNSs highlight the importance of clinical leadership and commitment to patients, nursing, and the organization. CNSs demonstrate professional leadership in their active participation in mentorship and empowerment to the organization by working on patient-care issues to improve patient outcomes and costs for specialty populations. Their role enhances others' perception of their value.

THE COSTS OF CNS PRACTICE

One key question for administrators is how to justify the cost of CNS practice. CNSs have done an excellent job of documenting the cost-effectiveness of their roles. The nurses and the institution benefit when length of stay is decreased; when complications of illness are prevented or recognized and treated early; when patients are satisfied and return to a practice or facility; when staff injury is prevented; when patients understand their disease and options for care; when cost-effective, safe, efficient equipment is selected and implemented; and when patient safety is addressed the patient. CNS cost-effectiveness is more than reimbursement from Medicare or an insurance company: it is often an intangible, difficult-to-measure benefit to their employer.

CHALLENGES TO CNS PRACTICE

Jones and Minarik[24] report on the plight of the psychiatric CNS, a role being challenged through a societal shift to Family Psychiatric Nurse Practitioner. CNSs are also being challenged by the Clinical Nurse Leader (CNL) role, the DNP, and the ignorance of the health care system as to the value of a multiskilled CNS in comparison with roles such as the single-skilled educator.

The CNL in particular has the potential to confuse the employer. One of the basic differences between the CNL and the CNS is that the CNS is regarded as an APRN whereas the CNL has been labeled an "advanced generalist." The APRN designation specifically includes medical diagnosis and management and prescriptive authority, whereas the hallmarks of CNS practice, such as integrating evidence-based practice into health care, designing programs of care and innovative nursing interventions, and providing leadership and education to nurses, are not expressly included in the CNL role. The astute employer would take into consideration the broad range of talent of the CNS, and get "more bang for the buck" when hiring the CNS in a hospital role.

Consider the typical nursing unit. The most valued leaders have always been the senior, highly experienced RNs. These experienced leaders know the systems, how to manage (or get around!) them, and where the power lies, and also know their patient population very well. CNS designation is the next natural step for these experienced RNs: education at a higher level in the specific patient population, with added benefit from education in medical diagnosis and management, advanced pharmacology, advanced pathophysiology, advanced assessment, research, quality improvement, teaching and learning, and evidence-based practice. The CNS can then support other experienced RNs with education, system interventions, and higher-level skills needed to make a unit run well with the ability to offer a very high level of care. The CNS knows the patient population, and can clinically assist the nurses with complicated patients, high-level assessments, and development of plans for care and related interventions. The CNS becomes the "go-to" nurse.

Not all states recognize the CNS as a protected title or as an APRN, which then, in those states, allows nurses to work in the CNS role without special education or certification. Hudspeth[25] sounded the alarm on the Consensus Model for APRN regulation and its impact on CNS employment. He noted that when the consensus documents are fully implemented, there will be a "large scale disenfranchisement of those nurses who hold graduate degrees in nursing, and who may have practiced in the role as a CNS for years, but who do not have any legal recognition allowing grandfathering, or who may be in a specialty that does not have sufficient numbers to maintain" a sound certification examination.

SUMMARY

The United States health care system is currently faced with many challenges, including access to care, providing high-quality care, and cost containment. The ACA is adding to the burden on health care systems in the United States by increasing the number of patients who will be attempting to access care. Accrediting agencies including the TJC, ANCC, and CMS expect that providers and institutions will provide safe, cost-effective, quality care to all patients. The evident needs of the health care system and expectations of health care consumers can be met by an exceptionally trained APRN, namely the CNS. Some stakeholders, such as the IOM, have already recognized the potential of the CNS in helping to address society's health care issues. However, nursing's contribution to role confusion related to the CNS, by developing competing roles that do not have APRN privileges, has created challenges for current and future CNSs to overcome.

This review demonstrates that the CNS is multidimensional as an independent licensed provider, expert clinician, consultant, and educator. CNSs in the United States have consistently documented outcomes including improved quality of care, decreased costs, and improved patient satisfaction. Health care in the United States needs individuals prepared to be agents of change, to improve current processes and outcomes, and to promote an environment of ongoing interprofessional assessment and improvement of health care delivery processes. The CNS is poised to help accomplish these goals.

REFERENCES

1. Dewitt K. Specialties in nursing. Am J Nurs 1900;1:14–7.
2. Hamric AB, Spross JA, Hanson CM. Advanced practice nursing: an integrative approach. 4th edition. St Louis (MO): Saunders Elsevier; 2009.
3. Bullough B. The law and the expanding nursing role. Am J Public Health 1976;66:249–54.
4. American Nurses Association. Nursing: a social policy statement. Kansas City (MO): American Nurses Association; 1980.
5. Institute of Medicine. Crossing the quality chasm: a new health system for the 21st century. Washington, DC: National Academy Press; 2001.
6. NACNS. A vision of the future for clinical nurse specialists. Harrisburg (PA): NACNS; 2007.
7. NACNS. Statement on clinical nurse specialist practice and education. 2nd edition. Harrisburg (PA): NACNS; 2004.
8. Hamric AB. Role development and functions. In: Spross J, Hamric AB, editors. The clinical nurse specialist in theory and practice. New York: Grune and Stratton; 1983. p. 39–56.
9. Fulton JS, Lyon BL, Goudreau KA. Foundations of clinical nurse specialist practice. New York: Springer; 2010.
10. CNAP. Texas needs a new approach to prescriptive authority. Available at: http://cnaptexas.org/associations/9823/files/CNAP%202013%20Legislative%20Initiative.pdf. Accessed May 6, 2012.
11. WOCN. Reimbursement of advanced practice registered nurse services: a fact sheet. J Wound Ostomy Continence Nurs 2012;39(Suppl 2):S7–16.
12. Institute of Medicine. The future of nursing: leading change, advancing health. Washington, DC: The National Academies Press; 2011.
13. Newhouse RP, Stanik-Hutt J, White KM. Advanced practice nurse outcomes 1990-2008: a systematic review. Nurs Econ 2011;29:230–51.

14. Arts EE, Landewe-Cleuren SA, Schaper NC, et al. The cost-effectiveness of substituting physicians with diabetes nurse specialists: a randomized controlled trial with 2-year follow-up. J Adv Nurs 2012;68:1224–34.
15. Muller AC, Hujcs M, Dubendorf P, et al. Clinical nurse specialist practice and magnet designation. Clin Nurse Spec 2010;24:252–9.
16. Gerard P. Reinventing the role of the clinical nurse specialist as practitioner-teacher to transform nursing education. Clin Nurse Spec 2010;24:277–8.
17. Charland K. Pay for performance comes to Medicare in 2009. Healthc Financ Manage 2007;61:60–4.
18. Tuite PK, George EL. The role of the clinical nurse specialist in facilitating evidence-based practice within a university setting. Crit Care Nurs Q 2010;33: 117–25.
19. Sedlak CA, Doheny MO, Jones SL, et al. The clinical nurse specialist as change agent: reducing employee injury and related costs. Clin Nurse Spec 2009;23: 309–13.
20. Moore J, McQuestion M. The clinical nurse specialist in chronic diseases. Clin Nurse Spec 2012;26:149–63.
21. Mahler A. The clinical nurse specialist role in developing a geropalliative model of care. Clin Nurse Spec 2010;24:18–23.
22. Hardie H, Leary A. Value to patients of a breast cancer clinical nurse specialist. Nurs Stand 2010;24:42–7.
23. Muller A, McCauley K, Harrington P, et al. Evidence-based practice implementation strategy: the central role of the clinical nurse specialist. Nurs Adm Q 2011;35: 140–51.
24. Jones JS, Minarik PA. The plight of the psychiatric clinical nurse specialist: the dismantling of the advanced practice nursing archetype. Clin Nurse Spec 2012;26:121–4.
25. Hudspeth R. Changes for the valuable clinical nurse specialist: a regulatory conundrum. Nurs Adm Q 2011;35:282–4.

The Honorable Arlene Wohlgemuth and the Texas Public Policy Foundation
Texas Treasures for Nurses

Cynthia Vorpahl Purcell, MSN, RN

KEYWORDS

- Advanced practice nurse • Affordable care act • Medicaid • ObamaCare • PPACA
- Policy • Wohlgemuth • Texas health policy

KEY POINTS

- Block Grants and Healthcare Compacts are potential solutions to the Medicaid economic crisis facing many states.
- Access to healthcare in Texas is significantly affected by limitations placed Advanced Practice Nurses in the State.
- The Texas Public Policy Foundation is a nonprofit, nonpartisan research organization, which provides credible information that nurses can use to influence health care policy.
- The Director of the Center for Health Care Policy at the Foundation, Ms Wohlgemuth, discusses the resources available.

Earlier this spring, this author had the honor of talking with the Honorable Arlene Wohlgemuth to learn more about the Texas Public Policy Foundation, the Center for Health Care Policy, and to discuss issues facing Texas, the nation, and Advanced Practice Nurses. The following article summarizes the conversation and information learned during the meeting.

Ms Wohlgemuth is the Executive Director and Director of the Center for Health Care Policy at the Texas Public Policy Foundation (the Foundation), a nonprofit, nonpartisan, free-market research institute based in Austin, Texas. She served the as a legislator for 10 years in the Texas House of Representatives specializing in health care issues, and has a well-documented track record in support of nursing, specifically expanding the scope of practice for advance practice nurses (APNs) in the State of Texas.

Disclosure of relationships: No relationships to disclose.
Dr Purcell is currently enrolled in the DNP program, University of Alabama, Birmingham, USA Department of Health Restoration and Care Systems Management, School of Nursing, University of Texas Health Science Center at San Antonio, 7703 Floyd Curl Drive, San Antonio, TX 78229, USA
E-mail address: purcellcv@gmail.com

Perioperative Nursing Clinics 7 (2012) 355–360
http://dx.doi.org/10.1016/j.cpen.2012.06.007
1556-7931/12/$ – see front matter © 2012 Elsevier Inc. All rights reserved.
periopnursing.theclinics.com

ABOUT THE TEXAS PUBLIC POLICY FOUNDATION

Founded in 1989 by James Leininger, of San Antonio, the Foundation is a $5 million research institute with a strong focus on conservative, free-market values. As a 501(c)(3) designated organization, the Foundation cannot be directly involved with, or participate in campaign or legislative activities.[1] The Foundation has 30 employees and 9 policy centers,[2] each with a specific mission and areas of focus (**Table 1**).

The overall mission of the Foundation is "to promote and defend liberty, personal responsibility, and free enterprise in Texas and the nation by educating and affecting policymakers and the Texas public policy debate with academically sound research and outreach."[2(p6)]

Ms Wohlgemuth was asked what sets the Foundation apart from other research institutes. She stated that whereas many think tanks and research institutes charge a fee for their services, the Foundation refuses to accept funded research. Their research is completely independent of financial or political influence (Arlene Wohlgemuth, personal communication, 2012). The work of the Foundation is used by local government, lawmakers, lobbyists, groups, and organizations in Texas (and other states) to inform policy makers on issues of economics, private rights, education, and health care.

ADVANCED PRACTICE NURSES IN TEXAS

Ms Wohlgemuth has been a staunch supporter of nursing and advanced nursing practice for many years. Policy analysts at the Foundation are convinced that Advanced

Table 1
Texas Public Policy Foundation centers and missions

Center	Mission
Armstrong Center for Energy and the Environment	"…Champions market-based stewardship of natural resources and provides principled solutions to environmental problems" (p. 10)
Center for Economic Freedom	"…Works to free citizens from interference in their private property rights and promotes a regulatory regime that enforces an honest, open marketplace" (p. 13)
Center for Education Policy	"…Provides market-based solutions to improve public education in Texas through school choice, competition, and greater spending transparency" (p. 12)
Center for Effective Justice	"…Works to reduce the negative human and economic impact of crime on victims and communities" (p. 14)
Center for Fiscal Policy	"…Advances prosperity through good stewardship of taxpayer dollars and promotes the principles of responsible taxation" (p. 7)
Center for Health Care Policy	"…Promotes a competitive private health care market with choice for consumers, lower prices, and improved quality" (p. 8)
Center for Higher Education	"…Champions a system of higher education with greater affordability, accessibility, quality, and transparency" (p. 9)
Laffer Center for Supply Side Economics	"…Cultivates the next generation of supply-side thinkers … able to articulate complex economic ideas in easily understandable terms" (p. 15)
Center for Tenth Amendment Studies	"…Works to restore the Constitutional balance between the states and the federal government" (p. 11)

Data from Texas Public Policy Foundation Annual Report. 2012.

Practice Registered Nurses (APRN) are a highly qualified, valuable, and critical resource in Texas and the nation. Ms Wohlgemuth reflected that sadly, Texas ranks as one of the most restrictive states in the United States with regard to APRN practice. In April 2011, she provided testimony to the Texas House Committee on Public Health in support of 3 bills that would expand the scope of practice for APRNs in Texas. She explained that in Texas, physicians are limited to a maximum of 4 nurse practitioners with whom they may collaborate. In the large urban areas of Texas, this is not necessarily a problem; however, many counties in Texas have very few, if any, physicians, and restricting each physician to only 4 nurse practitioners creates limitations on availability of health care providers.[3] Rural, isolated geography and financial constraints in many Texas counties have affected the ability to recruit and retain physicians. Additional restrictions that require physician practices to be no more than 75 miles from the nurse practitioner practice site further limit the number of health care providers available in these desperately underserved areas (Arlene Wohlgemuth, personal communication, 2012).

Research provided by the Foundation supports the role of the APRN in primary care and demonstrates the positive outcomes nurse practitioners have on health outcomes. Ms Wohlgemuth maintains that increasing the ratio of nurse practitioners to physicians and expanding the APRN scope of practice to the extent of their education would have a significant impact on access to health care in Texas, as well as an economic impact.[4] Economically, Texas struggles under the burden of providing health care through the Medicaid system. A great majority of Texans who live in areas with limited to no access to health care providers are also on Medicaid.

IS THERE A MEDICAID SOLUTION?

During the conversation, Ms Wohlgemuth expressed grave concern regarding the extreme economic burden placed by Medicaid on Texas as well as many other states. She emphasized that by the 2014-2015 biennium, nearly half of the budget for the State of Texas (46.6%) will be allocated for Medicaid (Arlene Wohlgemuth, personal communication, 2012). This dire economic situation is not unique to Texas; many states are facing the same burden of increasing Medicaid costs, without having freedom and control over administration of the system. As a means to stem the increasing costs of an inefficient system, the Foundation and the Center for Health Care Policy have proposed that Texas (and other states) seek "block grant" funding from the federal government to support state Medicaid programs.[5] She described a block grant as a source of minimally restrictive funding from the federal government. A block grant would allow a state the freedom to customize Medicaid programs and services to best fit the needs of their population (Arlene Wohlgemuth, personal communication, 2012). In the Foundation publication, *Medicaid Reform, Constructive Alternatives to a Failed Program,*[6] it is noted that block grants (federal funding with limited restrictions) would encourage new innovations and methods to decrease the costs and wastes of current Medicaid programs and increase the efficiency of the program, while also increasing access to health care for the millions of people on Medicaid. Coupled with less restrictive laws on APRN practice, block grants would potentially save money for the state while also increasing access to health care for its citizens.

HEALTH CARE REFORM

Statistics vary in regard of the actual number of the "uninsured" in Texas, but it is generally accepted that approximately 45% of the population has little or no access to health care. The combination of restrictive laws regarding APRN practice and the expansion of the Medicaid system under the Patient Protection and Affordability of Care Act (PPACA) will create an enormous need for health care providers in the state. It is estimated that the cost of providing care under the PPACA and an expanded Medicaid system will approach $30 billion for the State of Texas in the 2014-2015 biennium.[7] The Foundation has published numerous reports, presented informed debates on radio and television, and created a Web site (www.ppacaction.com) to inform the public of the impact of the PPACA on the Texas economy, small business, and the nation. While providing information on economic impact, the Foundation has also researched viable alternative options to the PPACA. One such option is the Health Care Compact.

When asked about the Health Care Compact, Ms Wohlgemuth explained that the compact, an concept originating from the Foundation and passed in the Texas State legislature in 2011, allows states that join the compact the freedom to craft their own health care plans and programs without hindrance from Washington, DC. To date, Georgia, Missouri, and Oklahoma have passed the multistate compact and several other states are considering doing so[2] (Arlene Wohlgemuth, personal communication, 2012).

Along with the Health Care Compact, another major work of the Foundation was the filing of 3 amicus curiae briefs with the US Supreme Court on behalf of the State of Florida, et al. in response to the cases challenging several aspects of the constitutionality of the PPACA. Ms Wohlgemuth described the 3 amicus briefs as some of the most significant work done by the Foundation to date (Arlene Wohlgemuth, personal communication, 2012). Although Texans are the primary population served by the Foundation, the impact and work of the Foundation is clearly beginning to expand beyond the borders of Texas.

CAN NURSES AFFECT HEALTH CARE POLICY?

Ms Wohlgemuth was quite emphatic when discussing ways that nurses and other members of the public can influence policy. She stressed that individuals should do whatever they can to develop a relationship with their state representatives and senators. When pressed, she stated that ways to develop relationships include working on a campaign, writing letters, calling by phone, and otherwise making oneself known (Arlene Wohlgemuth, personal communication, 2012). From the perspective of an elected official, written letters are more effective than email communication, because the sender has to take time and make a sincere effort to send the letter. In her experience, she considered one written letter represents an average of 30 to 40 people who had the same views but did not take the time to write (Arlene Wohlgemuth, personal communication, 2012). However, Ms Wohlgemuth conceded that an email correspondence was far better than no contact at all.

HOW CAN NURSES STAY UP TO DATE ON HEALTH POLICY ISSUES?

The nonpartisan, nonprofit nature of the Foundation and its research provides nurses with credible and valuable information that can be used to inform nursing practice and influence health care policy. The Foundation provides a wide variety of information sources and never charges for information.

- *Veritas.* Quarterly publication; provides special features on current activities and impact of the Foundation. A companion online version (with back issues) is also available.

- *TPP News.* Biweekly e-newsletter provided to keep readers updated on Foundation news; also includes timely information such as upcoming events.
- *Texas PolicyCast.* Weekly recorded audio policycast [sic], featuring conversations/interviews with "policy experts, issue analysts, elected officials and other opinion leaders." The policycast and archives are available on the Foundation Web site and the iTunes store (at no cost).[8]

In addition to *Veritas*, *TPP News*, and, *PolicyCast*, the foundation provides press releases, commentaries, and news clips to radio, television, and print media across the State of Texas. Each of the 9 centers publishes commentary and/or newsletters specific to their missions. According to the Foundation 2011 annual report, the foundation was "...featured in the media an average of 15 times every day."[2]

SOMETHING FOR EVERYONE

With 10 specific centers of focus, the Foundation provides excellent information on a wide range of topics, including health care policy. As an ardent advocate for nurses and nursing practice, The Honorable Arlene Wohlgemuth's prolific portfolio of essays, articles, interviews, and testimony on several aspects of health care policy provide concrete, valuable information to inform nursing practice and policy. To learn more about the Foundation and Ms Wohlgemuth, visit the Web site at www.texaspolicy.com.

SUMMARY

The Texas Public Policy Foundation is a nonprofit, nonpartisan research organization, which provides credible and valuable information that nurses can use in their pursuits to influence health care policy. The information is rich and is produced in such a way that the general public can understand not only the issues but also the impact of pending and future legislation. Their publications on the PPACA and issues affecting APN legislation and practice are excellent resources for nurses practicing in Texas, as well as around the nation. As the Director of the Center for Health Care Policy at the Foundation, Ms Wohlgemuth is an accessible and approachable resource and friend to nurses.

REFERENCES

1. Internal Revenue Service United States Department of the Treasury. Exemption requirements—section 501(c)3. Organizations. 2012. Available at: http://www.irs.gov/charities/charitable/article/0,,id=96099,00.html/. Accessed April 6, 2012.
2. Texas Public Policy Foundation (TPPF). Come and get it. In: Texas Public Policy Foundation 2011 Annual Report. Available at: http://www.texaspolicy.com/pdf/2011-AnnualReport-Final-posting-spreads.pdf. Accessed March 30, 2012.
3. Wohlgemuth A. Transcript of testimony before the house committee on public health. In: Texas Public Policy Foundation Policy Brief. 2011. Available at: http://www.texaspolicy.com/pdf/2011-04-20-testimony-ScopeofPractice-arw.pdf. Accessed March 30, 2012.
4. Young E. Testimony to the senate health and human services committee: relating to expanding scope of practice for advanced practice nurses. In: Texas Public Policy Foundation Policy Brief. 2010. Available at: http://www.texaspolicy.com/pdf/2010-02-testimony-ey.pdf. Accessed March 30, 2012.
5. Wohlgemuth A. Texas can lead the way on Medicaid reform. In: The Houston Chronicle 2012. Available at: http://www.chron.com/opinion/outlook/article/Texas-can-lead-the-way-on-Medicaid-reform-3354023.php. Accessed March 30, 2012.

6. Wohlgemuth A, Miller B, Harris S. Medicaid reform: constructive alternatives to a failed program. Austin (TX): Texas Public Policy Foundation; 2011. Available at: http://www.texaspolicy.com/pdf/2011-02-RR04-MedicaidReform-Constructive AlternativestoaFailedProgram-CHC-arw-bm-sh.pdf. Accessed March 30, 2012.
7. Wohlgemuth A, Harris S. Texas business and Obamacare. In: Texas Public Policy Foundation Policy Brief. 2012. Available at: http://www.texaspolicy.com/pdf/2012-01-PB02-TexasBusinessandObamaCare-CHCP-Wohlgemuth-Harris.pdf. Accessed April 10, 2012.
8. Texas Public Policy Foundation (TPPF). Ppacaction.com. Available at: http://ppacaction.com/. Accessed April 10, 2012.

Index

Perioperative Nursing Clinics 7 (2012) 361–365
http://dx.doi.org/10.1016/S1556-7931(12)00065-4
1556-7931/12/$ – see front matter © 2012 Elsevier Inc. All rights reserved.

periopnursing.theclinics.com

Printed and bound by CPI Group (UK) Ltd, Croydon, CR0 4YY

03/10/2024

01040457-0015